Praise for *Addiction—What's Really Going On?*

"Once I started reading *Addiction—What's Really Going On?* I could not put it down! You can tell the passion the author has as you read it. I can also tell how she learned about methadone and the patients as she progressed in her work. I am sorry we never had a chance to formally meet or maybe we did—I was at that National Conference she referred to and I am pleased that NAMA has been mentioned in the book."

Roxanne Baker, CMA, President
National Alliance of Methadone Advocates (NAMA)

"*Addiction—What's Really Going On?* is a red-hot page-turner, it is like reading about trench warfare. The authors lift the veil and bring light to our nation's underbelly. It is gritty and gripping as you enter the lives of those who are like crabs trying to get out of a barrel. This is the horrifying tale of what happens when you go down the river of substance abuse and you don't have a paddle. Hope comes when you realize that there are people in this world committed to unselfish service who have unconditional love for others. All people who work in this field deserve a national service medal. Thank you Deborah and Barbara for showing us your humanity and for what we can aspire to."

Anusha Amen-Ra, CNC, CEO,
Sacred Space Healing and Retreat Centers International, Inc.

"*Addiction—What's Really Going On?* is a truthful look into the world of Methadone Treatment with a mix of compassion and humor. It is a great read for those in the recovery field and provides insight for those who do not understand the life of addiction and recovery. Much applause to Dr. Sinor for bringing her friend's poignant story to life; a great tribute to Deborah McCloskey."

Lori Carter-Runyon, Executive Director
Hilltop Recovery Services

I0039447

"*Addiction—What's Really Going On?* is a page turner with a deceivingly simple point of view: A helper wanting to help and people needing her help, if only things were that simple. I am fascinated by this book on many levels. First, as a chemically dependent person in recovery; second, as an addictions therapist; and lastly, someone who simply loves a great read. As a person in recovery, the emotions, mindsets, and motivations of real people bound in the web of addiction are depicted in very realistic terms and empathically described right down to the most basic need for simple survival. As a therapist, I understand the balance between the desire to help and make a difference in the world and being at war with the realities of human, ethical, and bureaucratic limitations. I recommend this book to audiences in any helping profession, people in recovery, the families of drug addicts, and the users themselves."

Bill Urell, MA, CAAP-II,
Addictions Therapist for our older adult population
Author, *The Addiction Recovery Help Guide*

"Thank you for allowing me to read *Addiction—What's Really Going On?* This beautiful memoir is indeed a tribute to the humanity and dedication Deborah McCloskey brought to those suffering from severe addictions... you hear her voice clearly, as if she were right next to you retelling her powerful stories personally. The content has excellent crossover potential for professionals, lay people, and addicts alike because the individual stories of addiction ring true at all levels."

Laurie A. Gray, JD
Drug Court Intervention Program
Co-creator, Token of Change™

"While the description of the program setting and patients were, at times, quite grisly and depressing, *Addiction—What's Really Going On?* brought me back to my first week working in an OTP as a counselor... when I was handed a 150 patient caseload. The author's style is extremely compelling and the pages turned faster than all my other reading material. While the first four chapters may not warm communities to the idea of having programs in their neighborhoods, it still captures, for good or bad, the dynamic nature of the methadone treatment programs. Thank you for letting me read this important document."

Mark W. Parrino, MPA, President
American Association for the Treatment of Opioid Dependence
(AATOD)

"*Addiction—What's Really Going On?* is an authoritative, turbulent, and powerful book with a down to earth, gritty look into the dynamics of an inner-city methadone clinic's staff and clientele that offers a true, original, and confounding image of an underworld population rife with liars, thieves, and expert manipulators. The authors offer provocative psychological insights, such as how everyone is born to be addicted somehow; for example, how people always park their cars in the same place or go to work using the same route. Deborah McCloskey's skills as a counselor is also brought alive by the respect she achieved, and some of the questions she raises require our thought. Such as why are there commercials on television for medications (drugs) when there is supposed to be a war on drugs; or when will people get tired of paying for the reward of addiction at their children's expense; and, will they see the advantages of getting and staying clean and sober. This book is a testament that demands societal change, as well as, individual growth."

John E. Smethers, PhD
Author, *Scumbag Sewer Rats:
An Archetypal Understanding of Criminalized Drug Addicts*

Other Books by Barbara Sinor, PhD

Gifts From the Child Within (Second Edition 2008) Loving Healing Press; Ann Arbor, MI. www.lovinghealingpress.com

An Inspirational Guide for the Recovering Soul (2003) Astara, Inc.; Upland, CA. www.astara.org

Beyond Words: A Lexicon of Metaphysical Thought (Second Edition 1993) Astara, Inc.; Upland, CA. www.astara.org

ADDICTION

What's Really Going On?

Inside a Heroin Treatment Program

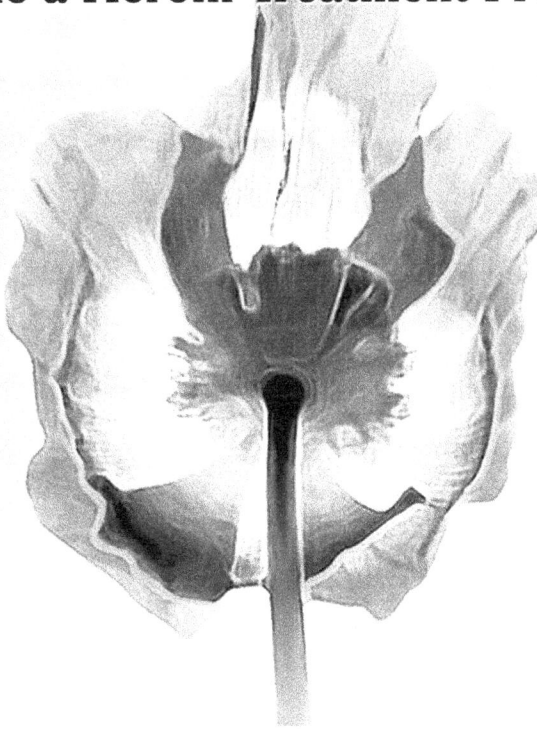

Deborah McCloskey, CADC
Barbara Sinor, PhD

Foreword by Mark W. Parrino, MPA

Library of Congress Cataloging-in-Publication Data

McCloskey, Deborah, 1954-2006.
  Addiction--what's really going on? : inside a heroin treatment program / Deborah McCloskey and Barbara Sinor ; foreword by Mark W. Parrino.
    p. cm.
  Includes bibliographical references and index.
  ISBN-13: 978-1-932690-93-4 (trade paper : alk. paper)
  ISBN-10: 1-932690-93-X (trade paper : alk. paper)
 1. Heroin abuse--Treatment--Case studies. 2. Methadone maintenance--Case studies. 3. Drug abuse counseling--Case studies. 4. Drug addicts--Rehabilitation--Case studies. I. Sinor, Barbara, 1945- II. Title.
  HV5822.H4M328 2009
  616.86'3206--dc22
                                                2009012983

Published by
Loving Healing Press   www.LHPress.com
5145 Pontiac Trail   Tollfree 888-761-6268
Ann Arbor, MI 48105   Fax 734-663-6861

CONTENTS

Dedication

I am sure Deborah would have wanted this book to be dedicated to her two amazing daughters, Jennifer and Lisa. These two young women were the center of Deborah's life. These successful young role models have developed into compassionate loving women like their mother.

Also, with Deborah, I want to dedicate this book to all those struggling with addictions of any kind. We encourage you to continue to educate yourself about the medication, alcohol, or drug which has controlled your life. Deborah and I ask you to find new directions, new possibilities for your life and to be gentle, yet persistent, in seeking addiction recovery.

Foreword

Treating addiction is one of the most complex things that any caregiver can do and it is also among the most richly rewarding. Consider what is done: An individual crosses the threshold of a treatment program or a doctor's office with the sense that a struggle has been lost and the individual is at the brink. When treatment works effectively with compassionate and knowledgeable caregivers, as depicted in this book, the integrity of the individual is restored and hope is rediscovered.

Addiction—What's Really Going On? is being published at a very challenging time in the history of opioid addiction treatment. While methadone maintenance treatment (MMT) has been used to treat patients with chronic opioid addiction in the United States for more than forty years, buprenorphine is a comparative newcomer during the past ten years. Both medications are extremely effective in treating long term chronic opioid addiction in a safe and therapeutic manner.

This book is also being published at a time of increasing and negative media reports about the use of methadone and associated mortality. This is driven by the increased use of methadone to treat pain in the United States. At the time of publication, there are approximately 260,000 patients receiving methadone maintenance in approximately 1,200 certified and highly regulated Opioid Treatment Programs (OTPs) in the country. At the same time, more than 700,000 patients receive access to methadone in pain management and physician office settings. We have also seen an enormous increase in methadone-associated mortality, which according to published federal reports, were outside the scope of the OTPs.

Addiction—What's Really Going On? captures the experiences of a clinician who worked in an OTP, then called a Methadone Maintenance Treatment facility (MMT). It is a compilation of personal experiences and observations. Some of the observations are not typical of the OTP experience, while many others are. It will be for the reader to determine what reflects the best aspect of patients being treated in OTPs and where there are flaws in a particular program's method of treating such patients.

Addiction—What's Really Going On? effectively captures the dynamic activity within the OTP and demonstrates the incredible relationship between the patients and the caregivers. Some caregivers, as depicted in this book, will be presented in an unflattering light while others continue to struggle against the reality of limited resources and the successful treatment of a complex illness.

There is a deeply personal and symbiotic relationship between the patient and the caregiver in these opioid treatment settings as noted throughout this book. While the content reflects one caregiver's journey in this rich and dynamic environment, I would encourage the reader to understand how complex the treatment experience can be. Not all the patients will respond effectively to treatment, but most will. A great therapeutic thread between a caregiver and a patient is what makes the entire treatment experience work. It affects the lives of the caregivers, the patients, and the families of both, to say nothing of the surrounding community.

From my point of view as an individual who spent nineteen years of professional life working in a methadone treatment program, both as a young clinician and later as an administrator, I can attest to the fact that working in a clinic is a life-altering experience. It was a favorable experience for me. It provides the caregiver with the privilege and the opportunity to work with extremely gifted patients who come from socially diverse backgrounds. It also gives the treatment provider the valuable opportunity to see how extremely effective medications such as methadone and buprenorphine can improve the lives of so many patients who cross our threshold.

I suspect that most will enjoy reading *Addiction—What's Really Going On?* while others may find fault based on their experiences. That is left to the province of the individual reader.

Mark W. Parrino, M.P.A., President
American Association for the Treatment of Opioid Dependence (AATOD)
March 2009

Introduction

We need to do more than just tell our troubles to God. God already knows. What we do need to learn to do is sit down with God and look for solutions: What actions to take, choices to make, directions to turn. In our conversation with God, we need to hear both the joyful and painful aspects of the situations in our lives. This is what I believe is 'turning it over.' Far from sitting and waiting for God to magically run our lives, turning it over involves turning in a *different direction*. Sometimes, that different direction is what allows us to discover and appreciate God in ways we never thought possible.

Father Leo Booth
Unity Newsletter July 3, 2003

A *different direction*, this is the message my dear friend Deborah McCloskey is clearly portraying throughout her engaging story. Deborah's untiring work to guide those in methadone treatment centers toward wise choices, developing self-esteem, and to search for new and different directions for their lives is obviously heroic.

Statistics tell us that the current need for addiction counselors, as well as rehabilitation and recovery clinics, far outweigh the current population need. In a paper prepared for the national Substance Abuse & Mental Health Services Administration (SAMHSA) titled "Substance Abuse Treatment Workforce Environmental Scan" it is noted that:

There has been a growing recognition that the substance abuse treatment field is facing a workforce crisis. Recruitment and retention of staff have surfaced as critical problems for many agencies as finding and keeping qualified professionals has become difficult for many administrators... Workforce issues are complex and woven into many issues facing the substance abuse field in general. Stigma, under funding, lack of resources, lack of public support, and misconceptions about substance abuse treatment affect the entire system, and of course, those who are employed in the field. However, the workforce is the underpinning of the entire infrastructure.

Obviously, the need for addiction and recovery counselors is paramount to the task of guiding those addicted to drugs (including methadone) and alcohol toward that *different direction* which can lead to a healthy sober future. Statistics from SAMHSA's National Survey on Drug Use & Health (2007) show there is an estimated 22.3 million persons over the age of twelve with substance dependence or abuse. This is almost ten percent of our national population. Although about 2.4 million people received treatment at a specialty facility in 2007, millions of others addicted to drugs and/or alcohol reported they needed treatment but did not receive help for their problem. More specifically, there has been no perceived change in the use of *heroin* over the last several years, 2002 to 2006.

Heroin is a chemical derived from one of nature's most beautiful flowers, the poppy. The specific poppy plant which yields opiates is the *papaver somniferous*. The production of opium and heroin from these lovely flowers was deemed illegal in the United States in 1920. However, stopping the underground drug market from smuggling the substance into our nation seems impossible. Heroin comes onto our streets from many countries including the Czech Republic, Mexico, Canada, Colombia, the Orient, and Southeast Asia. It is smuggled by air, sea, land, and even the mail.

Although heroin use may not hold the highest number of abusers over other forms of addictive substances—more than 600,000 in the United States—the social and health effects of heroin on our society is overwhelming. Family structures are compromised as jails are filled with addicted parents; education is impeded while children follow their family's substance abuse behaviors; and, our criminal justice, as well as, health and social services systems are all impacted negatively. Americans can now claim that almost half of us know someone with a substance abuse problem. I echo Deborah's puzzling question of "What's really going on in our society that we cannot deliver a workable and compassionate recovery program for our addicted population?"

Some feel methadone, a synthetic opiate, to be the best way to help those addicted to heroin become free of it. Others believe using an alternate addictive substance to achieve this freedom is a defeating measure in itself. Also, there is a common assumption surrounding the use of methadone that *once on methadone treatment always on methadone treatment*. In his acclaimed book *Recovery Options*, Dr. Joseph Volpicelli writes:

> Whatever the real reason for the perception, withdrawal is not the major obstacle to recovery: In the long run, staying away from street drugs is the real challenge... One study found that six years after detoxification following methadone maintenance, 83% of those who had been seen by themselves and by their counselors as ready to end treatment were heroin-free. Methadone maintenance does not have to last forever, although for some people, this might be advisable... Many people live full and productive lives on methadone, and many maintenance patients do withdraw from it successfully. Dead addicts, however, don't recover.

Despite methadone's obvious role in helping some heroin addicts, it does have addictive properties and, therefore, is also a risk for its user, its potential street market and the resulting social factors. On the other hand, methadone maintenance treatment programs (MMTs) are seen to reduce the risks associated with heroin addiction such as overdoses, HIV or hepatitis infection from shared needles, and to impinge a slight change on the illicit drug market.

For those proponents of methadone treatment, in the early 1970s MMT facilities expanded swiftly and were declared a success. Yet, growth of both MMT clinics and the numbers of patients treated quickly stagnated; then as now, MMT is available to only about one in five persons with... heroin addiction. ("Addiction Treatment Forum" Vol. 15, #3 Summer 2006) First, how can we in the mental health field guide those who want to rid themselves of heroin addiction by referring them to clinics do so if they do not exist? It is evident there is a need for more governmental, as well as, state and local social services surrounding all drug addiction facets when addicts have nowhere to go for direction in receiving care.

Dr. Vincent Dole who died at age ninety-three in 2006 was considered by many the "Father of MMT." He was highly respected for his *gentle giant* approach to patient advocacy. As you, the reader, will gather from unraveling the stories on the following pages, Deborah's counseling approach parallels that of Dole's who felt "...above all else, practitioners must *listen to their patients* to provide effective care." Dole taught that substance dependence "...is foremost a chronic, relapsing medical disease, rather than simply a moral, mental, or behavioral problem." These tenets held throughout Deborah's counseling career. We must not hold our addicted population to a personal moral judgment, but rather see and hear each individual as a soul whose life challenge is to stop abusing drugs and/or alcohol.

Deborah's counseling methodology was holistic in its approach. She openly confronted her clients as she would a friend or relative seeking her guidance. She used compassion, not judgment, while instructing her clients toward self-education, self-discovery, and self-recovery. These counseling methods both endeared her as "the counselor to get" and locked her into a decade of searching for better ways to help those she felt were stuck on the merry-go-round of a methadone system. She struggled, as many do, with the question of whether one addiction is better than another, for example methadone over other opiates. She struggled over heroin use passed from generation to generation among her clients. Deborah also struggled to introduce a compassionate and holistic concept of counseling by bridging the gap between labels and structure to one of caring and trust. She continually tried to devise avenues for her clients to rid themselves of their psychological dependence on methadone, therefore, releasing the need for lifetime treatment.

It is evident throughout this book that Deborah's passion for aiding those with addictions became her focus, as well as, to help redirect the way we as a society view and approach our drug addicted population. This passion led her to pose the compelling question: *What's really going on?*

At the time Deborah shared her writing notes with me so many years ago, I urged her to continue journaling her experiences and as the manuscript developed we worked together to form its balance between darkness and illumination. We shared our passion for client advocacy and discovered alternative ways to help those addicted to drugs and alcohol. I feel honored to complete her unfinished manuscript and bring her message of hope for a change in direction within the addiction recovery arena.

I have attempted to rewrite, edit, and gently interweave her powerful stories together, as well as, the immediate highs and lows of her own life to form a tapestry filled with pain, joy, defeat, and success. Although Deborah chose to call herself "Allie" in her journal notes, be assured the stories are true, the people are real, the life threatening incidents and tales of pain and death are factual. To balance the darkness of the addiction world, Deborah used her candid sense of humor which keeps you wanting to read what she will say or do next. You will search for illumination within the accounts of depression and defeat, but find it rarely. Only within a few select brave souls who have struggled to become drug-free will you find the answers to the book's questioning title.

Deborah continued guiding, counseling, and being a friend to her clients which she came to love until her death in 2006. I am proud to have been a friend of Deborah McCloskey and honor her work in the addiction recovery field. She was only fifty-two when she died, however, her decades of faithful diligence to her passion clearly declares that a *different direction* combined with *honest compassion* can be an answer to the addict's prayer.

Barbara Sinor, PhD

Genuine compassion is irrespective of
Other's attitude towards you...
But so long as others are also just like myself
And want happiness, do not want suffering,
And also have the right to overcome suffering,
On that basis, you develop some kind of sense of concern...
That is genuine compassion,
Now unbiased, even towards your enemy,
So long as that enemy is also a human being
Or other form of sentient being.
They also have the right to overcome suffering.
So on that basis, there is your sense of concern.
This is compassion.

His Holiness the Dalai Lama
From The Gethsemani Encounter, July 1996

1 Getting to Know the System

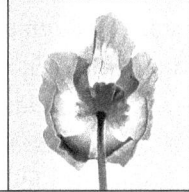

I do not think I truly understood the field of addiction until I had worked at the clinic for about six months. My parents, God bless them, were both alcoholics. I knew my clients did not exaggerate. I remember when I was sitting with my Father holding his hand in that damn hospital while he went through the DTs. I witnessed the various ways the patients were treated. Is it genetics? Is it social? Is it the foundation that you have or do not have? Is it the support systems? People in hospitals talk, always trying to discover why a person is addicted; the one my Father was in was no exception.

Dad never went to one AA meeting after his detox at that hospital, and he never drank again. He knew if he did, he would die. How could he just quit? He said, "Willpower." He was a regular guy, no special seminars, no Antabuse; he just used his mind-over-matter philosophy.

After my Father died and later with my first marriage, we tossed around the new diagnosis of "Adult Children of Alcoholics." My husband who was a workaholic, said our problems were all my fault because of my childhood with both parents being alcoholics. He found his excuse to not take responsibility within our marriage and rode it as a true victim. Our marriage was always in trouble. My husband was out of town five days each week. He once went to a therapist who also wanted to see me. The therapist's first comment was, "I understand you come from an alcoholic family." Was I the problem? Was my childhood destroying our marriage?

My cousin discovered 12 Step meetings and went to all of them. Did they help, or did she just find an easy way to make friends and fill her day while getting validation? I guess my family history urged me into school to study addiction and recovery. In the education program I attended, only two others claimed to not be an alcoholic or addict. The educational program I attended was located in southern California where I lived, it was a new program and we were the first class. The professor taught us all the basic psychological premises of alcoholism and addiction. He thought it was a choice to drink or use drugs and a choice to stop. "All in the power of the mind," he told us, "and a choice based on what options are available to the person." He had originally studied with Timothy Leary, or so he said.

The professor explained addiction as a temporary cure-all, "Any addiction starts as a fun escape, then goes to just an escape, and ends-up as a way of life. Boredom, guilt, regret, no sense of purpose, and most of all no self-love are the triggers for addiction." Also, he told us, "One needs to do something loveable to develop self-love." With these guideposts, we left school determined to help those with addictions find their self-love and move away from their unproductive and self-destructive lives. We had no idea what we were getting ourselves into! Thus, my life in treatment centers for substance abuse began...

~ ~ ~

"Oh, hi Todd," I answered the phone. "How are you? Still at that clinic? God, how do you handle the hours?"

Todd asked if I wanted to try a new job opening at the southern California clinic.

"Funny you should ask; I am looking at a stack of bills. My account balance says that is all I can do, just look at them. I haven't paid the rent on my Holistic Center for last month yet! I am going to close it soon. I guess running an alternative center just isn't my destiny."

He told me to drop by and meet the boss.

"Well, I don't have a current résumé, but okay, tomorrow at 10:00AM. Thanks, I'll see you tomorrow then," I told him.

It looked just as he said, a very plain two-story building completely unmarked, including the missing address. The windows were tinted and I would have missed it completely had it not been for the accurate description of nothingness and Todd's car out front.

"Glad you found the place," Todd said. "Come on in, let me introduce you to Javier. Allie, this is Javier, the Clinic Director."

"Hey Todd, can you give her an application? I'll be back later. Hey Allie, can you come back tomorrow?" Javier asked. "Ah, just call me tomorrow about this time."

"Sure," I said but silently thought so *glad I stayed up all night doing my résumé, spending fifty dollars that I didn't have on a manicure, copying all my certificates that validate I am worthy of your attention; oh, and thanks for leaving because I am a nervous wreck!* I stuck out my hand to shake, "Glad to meet you too, Javier. Todd has told me all about you."

"Wish I could spend more time with you now Allie, and yes, it is always this crazy. I will talk to you tomorrow. Todd, just leave her application and résumé on my desk. Thanks." And with that he was gone.

I spent the next three days playing telephone tag with this man. Todd told me it was a "sure thing." Sure enough, when I finally connected with Javier again, he simply told me to show up for work on Wednesday at 5:30AM.

I was strangely nervous. I could never have expected traffic jams at 4:30AM. The freeway was stopped and I did not know of an alternative route. My first day and I was late. It would take a lot of changes to get up at 3:30AM every morning. At least I knew someone who worked there, so I was not a total stranger. I wondered just what I would do there. It was July so the sun was just starting to rise and it was now 5:46AM. I could not believe that there was nowhere to park and I wondered why Todd had said, "Whatever you do, do *not* park in the parking lot."

I had lived just a few miles from the clinic several years before. In fact, I had shopped weekly at a nearby discount store. I had no idea that there was this type of clinic here, far less, heroin addicts inside. The building was a very plain two-story office building, close to several popular fast-food chains and a convenience store, right in the middle of a residential neighborhood. As I walked in the door a thick, sweet candy-like smell overwhelmed me. I struggled to place the scent, then it came to me. Once during class, my professor had said that methadone smelled like cotton candy; this smell was identical to his description.

The place was very active. People stood in line, most wearing sunglasses and all in various stages of dress with a variety of expressions on their faces. Most were checking me out in detail amid whispers of "that must be the new one," and a few cat-calls. Most just looked at me and pointed in unison to a space behind them in line. Everyone faced a set of windows, card in hand, urgently waiting their turn. I went to the counter that they were pointing to when I heard, "Are you private pay or MediCal?" The woman in the enclosed office did not bother to look up.

I said, "I am Allie. I am supposed to start working here today."

"How would I know that?" she said with an attitude. "Well, the Director is not here so I don't know what they want to do with you."

From behind me I hear, "Move it, bitch! I got things to do today."

I turned to face the dirtiest woman that I had ever seen standing behind me.

Most of her teeth were missing. Bright-red lipstick covered half her face, not just her lips. Her smeared eye makeup and unkempt hair looked as if it had been untouched for weeks. Her T-shirt was stained with various colors and apparently various substances. It was obvious she wore no bra and the spandex shorts may have been yellow once. Her legs had sores like swollen red-hot eggs and small scars that looked like cigarette burns all over, not to mention a couple of tattoo names on her neck, hands, and ankles. She wore very worn-out slip-on slippers, dirty purple. In fact, as my eyes remained at floor level, I saw most of them were wearing slippers! It was difficult not to stare.

She paid no attention to my paralyzed gaze and wide gaping mouth as she said to the lady on the other side of the window, "Give me my card." Then she walked away quickly to get her place in the line.

I was told to go upstairs to see a Todd, "Black Todd" they called him. Inside, there were two large staircases. The front of the building was crowded with people smoking and talking. Scanning the place, I realized there were children in the cars and more children outside tugging at their parents asking to leave. A sharp-dressed man directing traffic noticed my paralysis and asked, "Can I help you?"

I said that I was Allie, today was my first day, and I was to go upstairs to see a Todd.

"White Todd or Black Todd?" he asked. He pointed me in the right direction and added, "Oh no, gotta go. I'm Moses, glad to meet you." He turned to go outside, I watched him try to prevent one car from hitting another.

I started to walk up the stairs and my hand automatically went to reach for the guardrail when a voice from behind me instructed, "I wouldn't touch that if I were you, and watch your step."

I immediately removed my hand and looked up the stairs. I saw fast-food containers, beer cans, two cockroaches eating leftover nachos, and smelled an overwhelming stench of urine. The words "Oh my God," flew out of my mouth followed by, "A condom?"

"Get used to it. Hey, my name is Jack. Are you the new counselor?"

"Yes," I responded as I pushed my way into the door to get away from the smell. "I am looking for Todd."

"Black Todd or White Todd?" Jack asked.

Just then a man running down the hall said, "You Allie?"

"Yes."

"Did you bring any food with you?"

"No."

"Too bad, I'm hungry." I found out later that he was always hungry. He then said, "Your office is at the end of the hall, your charts are there, you can start reading them. Then you will spend some time with each counselor for their suggestions. See you already met Jack. By the way, I'm Black Todd."

I swear the only thoughts running through my mind were *how can anyone be hungry at this hour especially with these smells? and what am I doing here?*

"Glad to meet you," I said noticing that he never stopped moving down the hall as he continued talking.

The walls between the offices were paper thin; everyone had his or her door closed. My office was next to an outside exit and I had a beautiful view from my window. I guess you could call it beautiful, a Jacaranda tree with purple blossoms. Looking out the window, I could see most of the parking lot and swarms of people crossing the street coming to and leaving the clinic. This office location, I later learned, was a vantage for me.

I opened a chart but was stuck gazing out the window curiously watching all the people. I had never seen anything like this before in my life. It was like watching a movie, a cross between *Halloween* and *Night of the Living Dead*, only it was real life! Just then Todd (Black Todd) stopped at the door and announced lunch is in half an hour, and I would have time to go and introduce myself to Angie. *Where did the time go?* I wondered.

I walked down the hall and knocked on the door. This beautiful girl in her mid-twenties said in an angelic voice, "Yes, come in." Her office was like an oasis in the middle of hell with fresh paint and beautiful live plants. Renoir prints adorned the walls beside framed positive affirmations. Her hair and makeup were perfect. Her desk had closed charts mixed-in with a half-eaten bag of popcorn and a diet soda.

She looked up and said, "You must be the new counselor. I am Angie. How did you end up here?" She asked this question like my life had just taken a very dark direction. She picked-up a can of disinfectant spray and sprayed the room. Then she took an alcohol swab and cleaned her phone explaining that a client had just left her office. "Oh well, you'll get used to it," she said with a smile.

I started asking her questions, "How did you get here? How long have you worked here?" I looked out the window telling myself *Allie, you really need this job!*

Angie began a rant about the clients, not really a rant but a description with a tonality that emphasized her disgust with what the counselors had to handle at the clinic.

"You know most of them smell and most of the women have five to seven children in Foster Care *and* they are still prostituting. Oh, make sure you see Susie and get a lot of condoms, it is the least we can do. They are all on and off the system, you know, Welfare and Social Security. We have mothers and daughters on the program. In fact, I think we have one grandfather, father and grandson on the program! Three generations... well, the family that plays together as they say. Forgive me if I sound burned-out; my last client just told me she is pregnant, six months she says. How can women go around being pregnant and not know it, use drugs, and act like 'what's the big deal?' Now I have all this extra paperwork to do. Anyhow, it is lunch and I am starved. Do you want to go with me?"

"No, that's okay. I have errands to do," I lied. The truth? I was trying not to throw-up and to decide whether I really *did* need this job!

I went to my car and as I started to drive, I almost got hit by a client leaving the parking lot. People were everywhere. Later, I found out they were waiting for the next bus or waiting for the clinic to reopen.

My mind was racing. *Is this what I went to school for? Well, these are not bad people just sick people trying to get help, addiction is addiction. You only have to do this until the real estate market gets better. You can do this, it is only for a little while. How long has it been since you had a steady paycheck and benefits? Besides, you'll get off at 1:30PM You'll have the whole rest of the day! And you have bills to pay*! I returned to the clinic after lunch.

~ ~ ~

The doors to the clinic closed promptly at 10:00AM and opened again at 11:00AM. People who arrived late just waited in their car or stood in line outside the door for the hour if Moses was not there. The crowd in the afternoon did not compare to the morning crowd. The clinic was only open until 12:30PM because most clients needed to come in early before work so there was no need to stay open any later. Then the counselors had one hour to finish their chart work, doctor orders, or attend a meeting if scheduled. Then they could leave.

It appeared simple enough; one counselor had forty to fifty clients. If needed, a hold was put on their methadone dose until they saw me for fifteen minutes every two weeks which meant I would see a few of them daily. I would go over the treatment plan with them, write up notes, then go home and do it all over the next day. That is how my friend Todd (White Todd) explained it to me.

Todd worked a totally different job though. He worked with the clients that chose to sign up for the twenty-one-day detoxification program. I quickly learned that Todd did not have a clue what my job entailed, but later he found out.

I went home telling myself *I can handle this job. I am trained to help these people and they do need help.* "A steady paycheck and benefits" was the mantra echoing in my brain. *Mom always said I was to be a healer, this job is pretty close.*

Shifting my personal clock was not easy; I started my new job going to bed just about an hour before I was suppose to get up! I felt so sleepy driving home from the clinic but when I arrived, I could not nap. I quickly became extremely fearful of oversleeping, not hearing the alarm, and/or becoming very sleep deprived. Questioning my coworkers, I found that most took naps and went to bed at 8:30PM. My entire family, outside friends, and everyone else became aware of the person who must get up at 3:30 in the morning! It ruined my relationship with life. I could not stay up with the grownups, and frankly, I was too tired anyway!

The first few days, I think I drove to the clinic subconsciously. Sometimes I wondered *How did I get here? Was there a red light?* I drove surface streets through three cities before getting on the freeway due to the traffic. Yes, there was usually traffic this early in the morning. I had five more miles of surface streets before I arrived at the clinic. I became very conscious, no, more like paranoid of the cars on the road. At that hour of the morning as I got closer to the clinic, if a car close to me was not a late model with a recognizable coffee cup at the driver's lips, I wondered if it were a client on the way to the clinic or a drunken driver on the way home.

In fact, the city is a very strange world during the middle of the night. The number of people walking the streets at 4:00AM is alarming. They hang out at phone booths and laundromats. Some of them waiting on corners really do take the bus. Some of them are riding bikes. One thing that is really something to see is the number of people already in line at the Department of Motor Vehicles! Due to the clinic's odd workday, we became very isolated. At first, the jokes felt insensitive, cruel, sarcastic, and sick. But when we were handling the things we did at the clinic, we found comfort in our humor. We kidded each other that we would never fit into the rest of society again.

It was difficult to comprehend the choices these people made but then they had to accept such a distorted value system. At the clinic, we learned how to make the best of the limited resources and time, doing what we could for our clients while remaining professional. Not crossing boundaries was very important. The worst of it was trying to figure out whose side to be on: the addict and the damage done by "the system" or trying to work as a team with the various agencies— Social Services, Parole Board, DMV, Welfare, Child Protective Services, and Social Security.

2 | Getting to Know the Clients

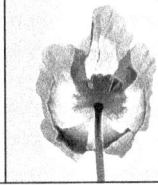

I had no idea when I arrived at the clinic that being client-friendly was automatic grounds for suspicion. I had always heard honey was sweeter than vinegar but I could feel the whispers, "She must be one of them, after all, who could be nice to these people." I was never sure which was more difficult, obtaining the trust of the clients or the staff, everyone was under suspicion.

Methadone clinics have had a history of problems surrounding them; drug dealing, drug diversion, cheating on urine tests, selling clean urine, it has all been done, not just at this clinic but at most. In fact, I learned that we had one of the best clinics and the most client-friendly around. Much to my surprise there were several methadone clinics nearby.

I do know that when I arrived at *this* clinic, I brought something that had been missing, perhaps a belief in humanity. Most counselors had been there for several years and the burnout was obvious. They were suffering from a constant internal challenge. They believed that all clients were manipulative liars, thieves, carjackers, murders, and prostitutes who were sucking-up tax dollars because of their habits, however, they deserved compassion, treatment, a kind word, and another chance. All the counselors had been *burned* several times by their clients.

I learned our Director was very compassionate but he would rule arbitrarily at the strangest of times. Nothing was ever clear-cut, ever. The rules for the clinic changed daily, or so it felt to me and several of the clients. The laws regulating methadone are always changing and the treatment is very closely documented. The uncertainty toward truth was a source of difficulty and fear was always present. I learned to work with instinct more than knowledge. The chemicals found in methadone are extremely dangerous. The average dose for a client could kill two drug-free people if consumed; however, we were not dealing with law-abiding citizens most of the time. Obviously, their histories shocked and amazed me.

We were very fortunate at this clinic, we had computers and a full-time doctor. Before I had started, everything had to be done by hand and it must have been very time consuming. The state and federal regulations required every milligram of methadone to be accounted for. All the bottles were numbered, all dispensing was recorded, and each client had a dosing history which included counseling attendance and urine test results. The date, time, and amount of the dose dispensed were recorded from each bottle.

Each client had to present identification at the dosing window, remove any kind of eyeglasses, and open his or her mouth wide so we could look for sponges or other drug diversion devices. Only then could they receive their dose. Before they could leave they must swallow the dose and then speak audibly, usually a "goodbye" or "thank you," to ensure that the medication has been swallowed. The client had to take this medication daily.

At the time I started at this clinic in the late 1990s, the census more than five hundred clients on the program with up to an additional one hundred in the twenty-one-day detox program. We had nine counselors, the Director, the assistant manager, two dispensing nurses, the doctor, one medical assistant, the detox counselor, and Moses for security. The bookkeeper, who was also the lady at the front window, had a job duty list too detailed to relate.

It was explained to me that the medication kept the addict free from withdrawal symptoms for twenty-four to thirty-six hours. I later found out this was true only in a perfect world. The biggest fear a client has is withdrawal. I cannot fully describe the panic, anxiety, and terror I observed regarding the possibility of this experience. An example would be when there was an impending bus strike, a client who had no money for a taxi, no other means of transportation, and could not walk to the clinic realized the limited hours the clinic was open. He would actually go into a cold sweat and need a counseling session just to make plans for how he would be able to get his dose that day. Then that client would start thinking of other circumstances, like what happens if we have an earthquake. In a panic he would say, "I don't want to use but I will if you make me. Most drug dealers will deliver you know?" I discovered this was true. It was in this type of situation when I learned the power of the brain, the power of words, and the power of trust. My clients, not my college education, taught me about addiction.

~ ~ ~

My first few days, I spent reading charts. The case notes all looked the same.

The treatment plans all looked the same. The only difference was the size of the chart and the initial clinical assessment. The assessment told me the age of the client when he or she first used, number of incarcerations, number of children, and so on. I was always amazed by client data; how old they were, how young they were, how little time in their lives they had been out of prison, the number of children they had, and how they got here. I later learned that the information was mostly unreliable. However, there was a lot of truth between the pages for those who cared to look.

The urine testing log was in the center of the chart. Each client had a mandatory random urinalysis every twenty-eight days. In my educational program, some of the students recounted tales of their own addictions but I was still so naïve. I mean, sure I had smoked some pot and I had taken a few cross tab whites (caffeine stimulants) when I was in school. I also admit to drinking alcohol but never had I seen, heard, or witnessed the variety of chemicals that this population smoked, snorted, ingested, or injected into their systems, sometimes in a single day! I was stunned by how many of these drugs were legal prescriptions, it was all in the charts! I never understood how the human body was so adaptable to all that these clients consumed.

The medication, methadone, that is taken daily (not forgetting that the average dose was strong enough to kill two people) was often washed down with a beer (yes, a beer), a few tokes off a joint, a Tylenol ™#3 or #4 with codeine, a Valium, or an eightball (a mixture of heroin with another drug) also known as a speedball, later in the afternoon. Then they were back in line at 5:30AM to start all over. And do not forget many clients also had legal prescriptions including antidepressants, medication for high blood pressure and diabetes, drugs for tuberculosis and AIDS, inhalers, and antibiotics. Of course, there were also those using methadone treatment as intended, to get their life together by getting off heroin. The only reminder of their past was that they, too, were forced to come to this location daily or weekly, a constant reminder that despite what they could establish, reestablish, or accomplish they were still one of *them* when they were here. Just my opinion.

I grew to understand that it was the fear of losing what stability they had been able to achieve that kept them returning to the clinic. It was also one of the few places they can go where someone would say, "Hey, Mary, how's the job and kids?" Maybe it was the only place they got a little acceptance, the possibility of respect, or normalcy. After all, they truly knew what they had accomplished. Yet they were fearful, no terrified, of forever cutting the cord for freedom from any drug, including methadone.

Now, the picture I have painted so far may lead one to believe that these folks are those in the back alleys, laying on benches in the park wearing overcoats, or movie stars from HBO's *The Wire*. Yes, some of them are like that. But most of our methadone patients were real mothers and fathers, clerks at grocery stores, the waitress at the coffee shop, the truck driver, the nurse in the hospital, the man who cleans your carpet, the person who sold you your car, the man who repaired your car, the lady in line next to you registering for the next cooking class, or the school bus driver. Real people, kind of scary, huh?

~ ~ ~

After one week of reading charts, getting aquatinted with the other counselors and the clinic procedures, it was time to get to work. I got the job due to the increase in census. This gave the counselors the chance to choose which clients they wanted to drop. Naturally, I got all the most difficult, most disgusting of clients. I received the ones who had been shuffled due to the level of difficulty, personality conflicts, the rule breakers or the ones that required effort, time, solutions, and baths. As Jack called them, "the high-profile clients." It was decided *for me* that the best way to meet them would be through urine testing. It would be on Monday.

I was learning how to set up the computer which put automatic holds on client doses and created labels and lists when I heard my name over the loudspeaker. A client needed to speak to me. As I walked to my office to get the client's chart, her ex-counselor stopped me and said, "She just lost her kids and that's all I have to say on the subject." She then turned her back to me and walked away.

It was totally unexpected to have a client request an appointment to talk to a counselor, far less to request a specific date and time. The current requirement was for thirty minutes of counseling a month and we practically had to force, take that back, we did have to force most of them to comply. This client said she had problems and she was desperate. Now with the clue that her ex-counselor just gave me, I could see why. She had no idea that I was her new counselor, so I went downstairs to introduce myself.

As I walked into the reception area the best description I can offer is there were chairs where we met our clients, at least for the first time. She appeared less than five feet tall and about eighty-five pounds at best. She looked about fourteen, but I knew better. Her long hair fell below her waist as she stood talking animatedly to another counselor.

I interrupted them, "Hi, my name is Allie. I understand that you need to make an appointment to talk to me?"

The other counselor quickly excused herself without saying another word. The childlike woman did not appear so childlike looking at her straight on. What was left of her makeup was smeared by tears, her face was expressionless. Apart from the tears themselves, I observed no emotion. Her mouth was moving but because I was so struck by the absence of teeth and the emotionless, tear-stained face, there was a delay in hearing what she was saying. Her hands desperately clutched her cigarettes and matches as she asked, "Can we talk outside so I can smoke?"

"Sure, it's noisy in here and I am having a hard time hearing you anyway," I agreed.

Her hands were shaking as she pulled out an already half-smoked cigarette. The clients often did this and it smelled worse than a fresh cigarette. I asked her, "What is your name?"

She began in a harsh tone, "Look lady, I had my kids taken away last night. Check my file, all my tests have been clean. I ain't never missed a day. I keep my trailer clean. I never leave my babies alone and I can't live without them. Look, my ex-old man and his woman can't make no babies, one phone call and she got mine taken. She wants *my* kids to hold on to *her* man. She said I left my babies alone for two days! I can't believe this is happening to me!"

I immediately remembered my first day at the clinic when Angie had told me similar stories. I felt the waves of nausea as I tried to control my emotions; they do not really train you for this in school. Of course, I immediately was gripped by client transference from my experience in divorce court when my ex-husband had tried to get custody of my daughters. It was so hard to stay present and fight back my tears. My client took a desperate drag on her cigarette saying she had to go because she could not miss her ride. Pointing to a car full of men, she asked if she could see me tomorrow.

"Yeah, but don't you think this needs your attention now? How old are your children?" I asked trying to get more information.

"Three and ten months," she said again glancing at the car now starting its engine.

"I can't imagine putting this off until tomorrow. Let's talk now," I offered. "You appear upset. Is there a social worker or someone we should call about your children?"

"I don't have no worker no more. I lost my worker when they took my kids last time. My sister won't talk to me, you know, she always has a bunch of guys over, they pay her. Ya know, rent money? But she told the manager that they were mine."

"Who?" I ask trying to keep up with the story.

"The kids," she says with an *aren't you listening?* tone to her voice. "Then they came and took them." She stopped talking and smiled. It was a mean, sinister sort of smile, smug-like.

Then she said, "It serves her right. My ex-old-man was so mad he left her. It's okay, my comrade has the kids now but she won't let me see them either. You know I spent money on them; I buy them what they need. Everybody said I was a good mom.

She glanced at the car, threw down her cigarette smashing it out with her slipper and said, "I have to go. They are going to leave without me. I'll talk to you tomorrow," she ended and got into the car which quickly left the parking lot burning rubber as it pulled out into traffic.

I stood there frozen, trying to sort my feelings from what actually happened. The counselor who she was talking to earlier came downstairs and put her hand on my shoulder and said, "Amazing how they can turn it on and off so quickly isn't it? I guess getting to her connection is more important than her kids now, huh?"

I did not even think about that possibility. As the counselor's words sank in, I fought my emotions and my denial and realized she had been the first client I had talked to at the clinic. What an introduction!

It was 12:30PM, time to lock up. I ran back up to my office and sat there trying to go over in my mind separating the words from what I had just seen. I tried shaking-off my experience with the threatened loss of custody of my own children, something I could not conceive living through. I tried to formulate a case note and started to review the chart. Tears were forming in the corner of my eyes when Jack stopped at my door and asked, "You didn't fall for her story did you?"

"What do you mean?" I asked him.

"Well, they get a new counselor and put on a real good show for a while, the concerned mother bit. You know the 'I am a victim' routine. Hell, she didn't tell you about her other five kids did she?"

The wave of nausea was back, "What do you mean, the other five children?"

"You haven't gone through her chart yet have you?" he asked with a smile.

"No, not yet. I am just trying to sort everything out for the case note."

"Well, you'll be getting a call from Child Protective Services in the next few days. Just make sure you have a signed release in there," Jack said pointing to the chart.

"Oh, I will. If there's not one already signed, I can get one tomorrow. We have an appointment for 9:00AM."

As those words came out of my mouth, Jack started laughing. "If she keeps that appointment," he said while walking away, "I'll buy you lunch for the next month!"

I thought to myself *What a bastard, doesn't anyone give these people a chance?*

3 | Initiation Day

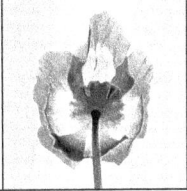

On the way home, I kept replaying in my mind what Jack and the ex-counselor had said about my first client keeping her appointment and talking with social services. We couldn't be certain she was going to her drug connection and that it was more important than her kids. I decided I could not take client stuff home, so I put it away until the next day.

The next day came much too soon for me and she did not keep her appointment. I checked the computer and she had dosed at 6:00AM. *I am sure she must have had a good reason to miss her appointment* I thought to myself. The counselors had been instructed to put a hold on a dose for all clients we needed to see—that was common practice. Jack, however, said he never did this unless it was urgent. He negotiated with his clients, "Don't mess with me and I won't mess with you." He also showed me how he used the window in his office as a vantage point.

Most of the clients were creatures of habit (no pun intended). They came at the same time every day, so Jack could see them walk or drive up and was Johnny-on-spot if he needed to see a client. "You can also watch for part-time employment," Jack stated. "You know, drug dealing or selling stolen items. I can also look into most of the cars and watch for dose diversion from my window."

Well, my new client had blown her first chance with me by missing her session so to make sure I did not miss her again, I put a hold on her dose for the next day. Maybe she was testing me, who knows, but I had to see how she was doing. Of course, I had projected all my values and feelings onto her by thinking how devastated she must be about losing custody of her children. What Jack had said about her other five children was true. I could not imagine having seven children, far less losing them all, but it was all there in the chart. Maybe she was making a new start for herself, maybe she was a victim, maybe I was *really* naïve.

~ ~ ~

I was sitting in the so-called reception area introducing myself to another client when I heard a woman's loud voice, "What the fuck do you mean there is a hold on my dose? Damn it, I am in a hurry. Call that goddamn counselor. I already saw her this week, what the hell does she want now? God, I hate it when they change counselors on you."

When the woman came around the corner from the dispensing windows, I saw that it was her, my client who had lost her children. I excused myself from my current client, I needed to talk to this screaming woman.

"Get the hold off my goddamn dose. I can't talk to you now, I gotta go. My ride is waiting and they will leave me here," she screamed.

"How is it going with your children? Did you talk to them or get to see them yet? Do you want to talk? I thought we had an appointment yesterday," I managed to get out hurriedly.

"Look lady, I can't be bothered now. Can't you see I can't miss my ride, I'll talk to you tomorrow," she sputtered.

Not even thinking that tomorrow was Saturday and I would not be at the clinic, I quickly removed the hold from the computer and said, "Take care."

She said, "Yeah, right," and walked quickly to the back of the line cursing about losing her place.

So much for counseling technique I thought.

I would have been offended if I had not heard this type of response before from other clients. In fact, it was sort of contagious—the "tantrum act out." If one client gets away with it, someone else tries it, then the group-bitching starts. "Yeah and you should see it in the morning, they think we have all day to wait!" Another one of the clients in line would start in, "And they never, ever open on time." You could see the patterns after a while and learn just where and when to draw the line, sometimes it was just better to let them whine. It often reminded me of school days, elementary school days, while we were all waiting in line for lunch. We do not have detention here but we *can* hold their dose.

About half an hour after the tantrum episode, I heard on the loudspeaker I had a call on line three. The woman identified herself as Sonja Johnson with the Department of Child Services and she wanted me to immediately fax my client's dosing records and urine test results. She stated she was certain there was a release in the file and that she needed the information immediately. In a sarcastic tone, she also told me she was aware that I was new to her client's case and she wanted to know how the counseling was going.

What Sonja really wanted to know was if I was able to complete a session with the client. I asked her if this call had anything to do with a custody hearing. Then I told her that, indeed, we had had a counseling session. The social worker did not have to know that I had gotten these facts in a two-minute, half-a-cigarette moment before she jumped into a car full of men, most likely headed for a drug connection.

"Oh, so you are aware that the children have been removed from her home?" Sonja asked.

"Yes," I responded politely.

Her response was quick, "Well, just get her records to me as quickly as possible." She gave me her fax number and hung-up.

I took the chart and the fax number downstairs. I had to take the chart apart to get all the documents and while filling out the fax cover sheet the clinic doctor walked in and peered over my shoulder. He picked-up the urinalysis report and stated, "She is not clean you know."

"Really?" I asked, "But the results all say she is clean."

"Yes," he said with a smile on his face, "but doctor knows."

"So, do you want to share your secret? You know I am new to this game."

"Look here," he pointed to the chart, "When we took her on as a patient at the clinic, her physical weigh-in was one hundred and fifty-eight pounds. See her picture? All the clients at the time of intake get two Polaroid photos taken, one for the office file and one for the identification card for dosing."

She had lost so much weight, it was hard to imagine it could be a picture of the same woman.

The doctor continued to suggest that I surprise her with a urine test. "I bet you, she is using some form of methamphetamine. In fact, why don't you test your entire caseload, it does them good to be surprised sometimes."

"I have already scheduled testing for Monday," I said.

"Good, you can handle it then," he reassured me.

I asked him about the reports, "Should I still send them?"

"Why not? We can't prove what we think." So I faxed the requested documents to the social worker with the attitude.

~ ~ ~

I had no idea what I was in for with the urine testing. Of course, the staff was very helpful and cooperative. They setup the computer, showed me where the bottles were, went over the rules of the observation room, as well as, how to send off samples to the lab. It did not seem like it should be big deal, I was not even disgusted at the idea of collecting the urine. To this day, I can still recall its smell, it is a dark brownish-orange thick smell, acid-like. The ventilation system was poor and the air conditioners overworked due to the doors being left open. Also, a heat wave was hitting a hundred degrees plus that day.

The acid-like smell lingered in the air along with the stench of those who had held their bowels to let loose while there. Well, you could smell it all the way out the front door. It was like the only revenge they could act out without anyone doing anything about it. Some of them jammed the toilets or stole the paper. We had two toilets and tested about one hundred people a day, often within two hours. It moved fast and went anything but smooth. Many times, I did not know which smell made me gag the most. That was one thing about the clinic, there were always strong smells present.

The building housing the clinic was next door to a fast-food restaurant. Within the first week, I learned there was a problem with rats in the attic. Remember, this was summer in the middle of a heat wave. I became the *authoritative nose* and was correct too many times. Often, Jack and I were the first to open the upstairs in the morning and there would be a faint whiff of something that grew stronger by the hour, a smell I quickly learned to identify. There must have been a better solution than rat traps which leave the animal dead for possibly several days before discovery. Another part of the uniqueness of working in the clinic, I figured.

One of the counselors had given me a word of caution, "It would be a good idea to be early on Monday. You know the natives don't like surprises."

Well, I took the advice and was there a good fifteen minutes early. I had my client list and all the bottles set out. I made a pot of coffee, got my computer set up, and had the gloves out and ready. It sounds like I was ready, right? No one could have prepared me for what was about to happen.

I still did not have all the faces and names matched, which only added to my problems. Some of the clients had been on the program for years. I could read their thoughts, "The least you could do after nine years of coming here is know my goddamn name."

I, myself, had never been urine tested. I had never known anyone who had to do it either. I had no idea what to look for in cheating on such a test, how to catch them cheating, or how to handle it if I did! Again, textbooks don't teach this.

The usual fifteen to twenty people were already in line pounding on the front door. The clock read 5:25, we opened at 5:30AM. Various statements were shouted-out and were reminders of how busy *their* day was and how our clocks were always wrong. "Hey, are you testing today or what?" kept ringing down the line.

I had no idea this was *my* initiation day today. Testing day was when I saw all my clients on the same day. I learned how to incorporate every skill in customer service; humor, BS, or whatever it took to get me through this day. Trust me, I learned real quick what name went with what face. The doors opened right at 5:30AM and they stormed-in. Some had their personal ID cards, some had to get their cards at the window, but all of them ended up in line for dosing.

I had officially met very few clients so far and none of them were in line. I was told about a few clients who were known to cheat on their test and to observe them. The best advice I ever got was from Angie, "Do not ever, ever, lie for a client; cheat for a client; or, try to cover up a mistake. If everything is upfront, there is a way to correct any mistake. With approval, the rules can often be bent but clients have no loyalty."

It was so hard to tell when I was being conned. I have always been honest around seemingly honest people and lived a fairly sheltered life. I was amazed at what people will do to survive. I witnessed many just trying to hold on to their world with the slightest bit of control. I was told one day when we were reflecting on client stories that a con cannot be an asshole, he has to be likeable. He has to hold your attention to get what he wants. You cannot piss-off a mark, or you lose the mark—the new counselor is always a mark.

I had a clear view of the dosing window from the testing room when I heard, "What do you mean I have to test first? I just tested last week!" So goes the first con.

"Hey, I have to get to work, can we do this tomorrow?"

Well, it sounded legitimate, so I said, "Let me go see." I went to find his counselor. I did not know he was laughing at me.

"Jim, give her a break," was the next thing I heard. "Just get in there and piss." It was Jack talking to the client, so Jim took the bottle and went into the bathroom.

I went into the observation room, no one told me to turn off the light. The client said, "How about a little privacy, bitch." I walked out and closed the door. He presented me with the urine sample immediately.

I cleared him and said, "Thank you." He got back in line like a lamb.

The next client took the bottle and said, "Cm'on baby, wanna watch?"

I was disgusted and embarrassed but managed to say, "No, thanks. Maybe next time."

The next woman started to con me, "Gim'me a break, I got three kids I gotta get to school and I am on my period."

Well, that made me think as I answered, "No, sorry. Come on, you know the rules better than I do."

Sometimes we would get a cold piss which obviously was not fresh or a really hot piss when clients put their sample into a microwave before coming to the clinic. Some clients, much to my surprise, went home and called other clients to tell them I was the one doing the testing. I learned about selling piss, getting your children to piss, and everything about piss. Also, I learned how hard it is to piss when you are on methadone. But the rules state always come to the clinic prepared to piss, this was the only consistent rule.

~ ~ ~

Out of all the challenges in life that present the opportunity to excel, I took pride in being great at urine testing. One needs to be great at something, right? Okay, I know there was the smell and the lack of dignity, however, I turned a crappie job—I mean a pissy job—into fun. It was a humiliating job for most, time consuming and disgusting. If I had to depend on urine testing for treatment progress, I was in trouble. It was performed more for program compliance to make sure there was methadone in the client's system and, of course, data accumulation for the agencies. It was also the method that kept tabs on what the drug of choice happened to be for the month.

For each of the sarcastic statements dished out, I soon created a comeback: "Yeah, yeah, I know you pissed on Tuesday but I have a black market and a girl has to make a living" or "Look at your thing? Give me a break, this is a professional you're working with" and "I can tell by the shape of your mouth if you're urinating or not." This last comment shut up one client. When he came out of the restroom, he asked me if it were true!

"Yeah, you look like this," I said squinting my eyes and making a wide closed-mouth grin. Everyone that was standing in line cracked-up with laughter.

My reputation had begun. I was (a) client friendly, (b) not easily rocked or bullshitted, and (c) had a sense of humor. I do think you can tell if a man is legitimately urinating by the look on his face. And I swear to you, I never looked at or saw a client's *unit*.

Some urine samples were collected *after* they had been standing in line and their dose had cleared. I would walk up to them, motion for them to follow me as we stepped aside from anyone who could hear and I would whisper, "Don't ever try to cheat again, or you will be sorry." I would never get cold piss from that person again.

Then there was a sample bottle so hot that I dropped it when I touched it. Not to worry, I did not spill a drop. I confronted the seventy-two year-old man who handed it to me, "Hey, what's up with this? A micro-piss?"

He said, "I'm so, so sorry, but I can't go and I can't hold up my ride. I have no way home. I didn't know what else to do. I am so ashamed."

I mean, come on now, this guy was seventy-two frigg'n years old! He was dressed nice and was clean looking, so I told him we would discuss it in our next counseling session and I expected to see him when he got there tomorrow.

"Yes ma'am," he said, "Thank you ma'am, permission to go back in line ma'am."

I swear he was being honest from the depths of his soul. I found out later that he had been.

So, is this enabling, cheating, giving them a chance? Whatever it was, it was my style, my method. Sometimes you have to think quick, get to the best solution for all involved and still remain legal. I quickly learned to separate those with truth and those with stories. Opportunities to be a jerk or pull out your power card were endless, but it was just as easy to try to get along with the clients. Remember, being on this program was a choice for most of them, if they really did have a choice.

During test day, I also got to meet all the clinic's clients. I was not sequestered in my office but out in the front office, the front lines. This is where *I* got tested, not just by my clients but all of the clients. They checked me out thoroughly, "Hey, nice wedding ring, you wanna sell it?" "Hey lady, you use too?" "You look tired this morning, party last night?" Always with the sassy comments! I also ran into hustlers with something to sell. Of course, we are not allowed to purchase anything or accept any gifts.

I learned this clinic was different from most. It was what they called a *family clinic*. Most of the clients lived nearby. They were not transients as in Hollywood where they got so many street people. At this location, we have wives paying for husbands and husbands paying for wives; husbands and wives together; aunts, uncles, cousins, sisters and brothers all heroin users, a real family affair. Grown men living at home with their mothers was one of the most common social dynamics. The mothers paid for their son's clinic visits even though many of these "boys" were in their fifties.

| 4 | Methadone: Pros and Cons | 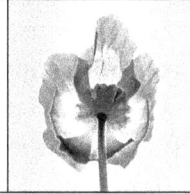 |

Test day was always more of a test for the counselors than the clients. Would there be enough bottles? What would the weather be like? Who would be the jerk of the day? Many clients stood around because they could not urinate, they would drink lots of water but I give them coffee. Methadone can effect constipation, urination, and for some, impotence. The other thing I did was to actually look at the urine sample and offer a kind word, "Hey, Joe I think you should be drinking more water" or "Hey, we got some information about Hepatitis, remind me to share it with you next session."

All the clients had an initial physical examination when they came on the program and annually thereafter. Hepatitis B and various forms of Hepatitis C are being discovered in ninety percent of the clients at clinics which distribute methadone, not to mention tuberculosis (TB). We had to screen for some very nasty diseases. We were required to monitor their health, follow up on all prescribed medications and future medical/dental appointments. We were actually powerless with most follow-ups, but I found a way to manipulate some of the clients by using a doctor across the street which worked with me to help them stay healthy.

Doctor prescribed controlled substances were one of the worst problems, it was a tough call most of the time. Due to a drug overdose death, our clinic physician no longer approved client prescriptions for codeine, or any prescription that included codeine. Codeine is a drug that communicates with the brain that controls the cough and pain centers. Methadone does not alleviate pain. Many of our clients had several physical disabilities and together with their high tolerance for drugs and frequent abuse of medications, it took a lot of drugs to make the hurt go away.

Addicts have pain too, in fact, a very low tolerance to pain. This fact may be why many of them ended-up at the clinic. The local area doctors gave out prescriptions for codeine like peppermints. It was a constant source of trouble. One woman who came to the clinic took an average of sixty pills a day, she wanted our help in sorting them all out. It is amazing how she was able to get them all, far less, that she has a stomach left!

If a prescription was not approved and the client took the medication, it appeared in his urine test. Hospitalization with needed documentation was the only other choice. If there were agencies involved, like Child Protective Services or the Parole Board, it meant the loss of freedom or children. We also had a program where clients, if approved and criteria met, could get take-homes. When this happened, the client earned the right to not come to the clinic for a day or even up to one week. If they had a *dirty* urine test, this choice was not possible.

We gave take-homes for the holidays. Many times, a client would get the flu in November and his medical doctor would give him Fenesin™, a cough syrup containing codeine which was not cleared. Subsequently, many needed to be at the clinic on Christmas day and New Year's morning. So you can imagine all the difficulties, as well as, the desperation in their pleas and efforts to prove their worthiness of a take-home. How do you explain to unknowing family members of your disappearance at 7:00AM on Christmas morning?

We did get our doctor to lighten-up a little but the real problem was the other physicians caring for a client. They gave the same prescription over and over, thus creating another addiction and a real problem; treatment versus treatment and doctor versus doctor. I quickly became a believer in alternative medicines and so did some of the other counselors.

Since most of the clients were from this local area and on MediCal, we saw the same physician names over and over again. We could easily tell which physicians were the "script-writers." Let's face it, when clients do not have the best medical care, they do not care. If they are not interested in medical care, it is not difficult for them to get the medications they want on the street market.

I should also mention that the current street price for a pill like Valium or codeine was usually two dollars, unless you had some spare change and a cigarette or two. I have never understood why a computer cannot track and/or trace prescriptions. How do you argue this need? We kept trying to argue this point at the clinic.

Once when we had some extra money in the budget, so we decided to hand out a multivitamin tablet with each dose. It was optional and we thought we should try to help the clients meet dietary needs. This goodwill gesture became a source of humor.

One time a client called me downstairs and said, "Hey, I am addicted to those things they have been giving me and now they are out of them! What am I going to do? What are they called? I get a good high off them." He was a clown, of course, but again it was finding the humor in the little things that helped keep me conscious.

It was optional, but we were lucky to have a person from the county to help us with AIDS education and testing. The education was mandatory, we were trained to provide the necessary information but we just supplemented. It was better to have Susie do it, she could often get them to open up more in that area than the primary counselor. The clients wanted to appear stable with the clinic counselors.

Susie would get all the good gossip, hand out condoms, and get them to take an AIDS test every six months if she and they thought it necessary. The greatest invention for our clinic was the oral test for AIDS, many of the clients refused testing for a long time because of the difficulty in locating veins for a blood draw, now it is like a lollipop, ah progress.

Susie's office was in the center of the other offices, what a shock one would get when the door was opened. Every type of condom imaginable was posted on the walls! Companies and individuals from all over the world sent them to Susie, also dildos in various shapes and colors. On top of that, there was a stain on the ceiling tiles from one of the rains that I could swear was the shape of a penis!

When we met, I found it funny and somewhat embarrassing that, no, I did not know how to use a condom. This topic became one of my required classes which I gave to clients just to make sure that *they* knew. After all we had seen at the clinic, as well as, the pictures from the county and considering all the trust factors, I marched home with quite a collection of condoms one day. My husband asked, "What the hell are these for?"

"Never mind," I said.

But when his son went off to college, I wrapped up all the condoms in a basket filled with a full set of disease photos and a card that read, "Friends don't let other friends have casual sex without protection." I just hope the photos made him reconsider, they made us think. Actually, the photos were enough to take away any thought of physical desire!

~ ~ ~

The counselors had to take turns once a month to work the weekend, since I was the new kid, I got the opportunity the third week after I started. I was just getting over the initial shock of working in the clinic. Nothing could have prepared me for Saturday and Sunday mornings. We opened at 7:00AM and closed at 9:00AM. As I pulled up, the line was twice as long as usual and it was only 6:45AM. I had to take cash from the clients on the twenty-one-day detoxification program and give out their cards. This was not a problem, except we never seemed to have change.

The *fee detoxification* program was something I had not yet learned about. This program was when a client was on a monthly maintenance program and paid privately. If he did not pay, the client was forced to detox. The only insurance company which I was aware of that paid for methadone was MediCal. The cost was two hundred dollars per month. If a client was unable to pay, the dose was reduced by the number of milligrams it would take to get them to zero milligrams in fourteen days. As soon as they could pay, the dose was reinstated the next day, if approved by the doctor. On Saturdays, *if* the client could pay, *usually* the doctor could be contacted by phone and the dose was given, however, there were often circumstances when this did not happen.

Many client stories went like this: "You'll be forcing me to use" or "I have a job and I can't afford to be sick" or "How can you do this to me after years of loyalty?" The truth was if they took the time to make the payment arrangements things could have been worked out. However, there were clients with their bill so high it never could be worked-out, and of course, it was all our fault.

Then there were clients that disappeared for a week or more, a *no show*. After fourteen days of no shows, they were automatically discharged. If they were a no show for more than three days, they had to be reinstated by the doctor. If a client had a string of no shows, all the agencies automatically assumed he is using again. "I *need* my dose," I would hear and I believed they really did. How could we make them understand it was *because* they skipped a dose that they felt so bad?

Then there were the clients that got arrested. Only one of our local police departments learned that their lives truly were easier if they got the client/inmate their dose while incarcerated. Escorted in by two officers, the handcuffed client humbly takes the dose and gets back into the car. They seem extremely grateful for the generosity of the officers.

If clients were arrested and in the county jail, they could be dosed by only one treatment center, not the clinic. The fees had to be paid with cash in advance for dosing and it was twice as much money as in the clinic. Also, the office that took the cash payment was not in an accessible location. But the real problem was they could not call their uncle Joe to come in and pay for them either because the records at the clinic were confidential. We could not verify the dose because we could not verify the client was actually here. It was impossible to have a blank, signed release in the file. Complicated enough? Three-way calling often helped, however, another problem due to these circumstances was the clinic never accepts collect calls which was the only call one could make from jail, if they let you.

~ ~ ~

So the doors opened at 7:00AM and, of course, they are all in a hurry. My jokes at my "inability to perform on the spot" were barely tolerated, the clinic being an equal opportunity employer and all. I had established myself and gone without enemies to date but that did not last.

The various stages of dress for the clients on the weekend made the weekday mornings look boring. I discovered we were hosting the Boulevard Girls, a local street known for hookers, and many of them were our clients. I quickly learned to make sure to grab a box of condoms from Susie for the weekend handout on Saturday and Sunday mornings. She never did stop asking me about my wild plans for the weekends, well, I guess a box of condoms is an unusual request. The clients arrived in pajamas, robes, party dresses, whatever. Pride was not an issue, fashion was not an issue, just the dose.

It took me awhile to understand that alcohol and methadone do not go together. The synergy of the chemicals in a body's system and the effect of alcohol on the metabolizing of the methadone just do not mix. Seriously, it was a very big problem for many reasons, not to ignore the obvious. First of all, the breath of a party animal first thing in the morning was enough to knock you over. If a counselor had been drinking, he could not smell the alcohol on the client; if the counselor had not been drinking, he could not escape from it here.

My own theories are that the body's system with methadone does not metabolize the alcohol as quickly. The other problem is something we do know, that alcohol metabolizes the methadone faster, thus, the withdrawal cravings kick-in sooner. It took me awhile to connect the facts, there are no mysteries, just science and someone caring enough to put two-and-two together.

Many times we would have to utilize a breathalyzer to determine the level of current intoxication before administering the dose. Sometimes clients had just left a party to come to the clinic. If their level of alcohol was too high, we would refuse to give them the dose. During the week, they could always come back in the afternoon which gave them time to sober up, but on Saturday and Sunday this was not possible, so those clients were not happy campers.

The tool that eventually aided my efforts in alcohol abstinence was the information I obtained about Hepatitis C. The few clients with this diagnosis that were still on the program helped me in my efforts to increase the awareness of what drinking alcohol while on methadone does to the human body.

~ ~ ~

Monday mornings were typically for prescription approvals or dose adjustments. Dose adjustments took time to understand. If a counselor did not take the time, the alternative was to just give them what they want. Initially, the doctor determines the dose based on the client's stated amount of heroin use. Working with the client's dose to get it right took effort and understanding. I do not mean to pat myself on the back or anything but like any medical mystery it takes two, the patient and the healer.

Our clinic physician would start most of the clients at 40 to 60 milligrams which should be enough to hold most addicts. But due to the extent of many of their habits, they may need more to start out. In one of my education sessions, an old-timer, a client, taught me about *their world*. What better teacher than someone who helped get clinics open years ago? She stated that anymore than a 40 milligram dose was just to get high, or they were still getting high. Since the average dose was 80 milligrams, I kept that fact in the back of my mind.

We human beings develop a tolerance to most any chemical in our systems and some clients truly did need a higher dose than normal. The rule was that if a client had evidenced drug use to automatically increase the dose, this did not work in real life. This guideline may apply if the client was committed to being free from any drug use and the medication did not hold them. But then many would go out and use heroin just to get stable. Not once did I meet that type of client, well, maybe once. I think most were just testing themselves, or the methadone.

One common thought at the clinic was that the clients liked to manipulate their dose for the *feeling* and that they would intentionally request a dose to be high for the effect. When they no longer received the effectual feeling, they would lower it for a while then up it again to get the desired effect. I did not run into that profile often either. The most frequent dose abuser was the individual who knew he would go on fee detox. He would raise his dose so the eventual declining dosage would not affect him as much. He knew when the bill would be paid, it was also a way of justifying his once a month use.

An alcoholic client would never have a stable dose as the methadone washes out of the system. So of course, with some clients my first question would be, "Have you been drinking?" The other common thread I found was with women who still had their menstrual cycles. For the ones that were clean, PMS was real and once a month they would request a dose increase unsure of why it made them feel better. Then I suggested it was PMS. It seemed simple enough to deduce but no one had taken the time to explain this to them, even though some doses for these women had risen to the 100 milligram range.

The highest dose any of us had ever seen was 180 milligrams. It was inconceivable how this client could function on that high of a dose. I later discovered that out-of-state the doses were much higher. The 180mg. dose client wanted to transfer from somewhere to our clinic, but there was no way we could accommodate the high dose either morally, ethically, or legally.

Outside laborers posed another problem. When the heat hit 100 degrees and they were working in warehouses or on construction sites, the methadone would sweat right out of them. Of course, the beers with the boys would have to stop. Then there were the clients that used methadone to keep the heroin habit lower so they could manage the addiction. They had no intention of quitting, the habit was just not affordable. Then there were the crack users which were difficult for me to watch. The crack, like alcohol, eats up the methadone along with their teeth, bones, and soul. I might add that the crack users were not very nice people either.

Once we went through a run of eightballs or speedballs where they mix heroin with some sort of crack, cocaine, methamphetamine, crystal, or speed. I asked my clients to explain this to me. They said when the heroin was of such poor quality, they had to mix it with something to get high. Another good line was, "I like the feeling when I am mellow but with a buzz."

Listening to our doctor try to explain an eightball sounded so funny. He would ask, "Tell me again, you take one to get high, one to get low, so you spent all your money to feel normal? I don't understand!"

We later discovered through the clients that most of the drug dealers were setting up new markets. If heroin was the drug of choice, then you got free crystal meth; if meth was your drug, then you got free heroin. It was called marketing strategies. Today, heroin use is on the rise with our teenage girls, the lowest prices in three decades and I hear the quality is good again.

Some clients took a long time to earn their trust, or you had to drag the information out of them. Most of the medications for AIDS and TB seriously deplete the effect of methadone. These clients would not take their prescribed medication because it made them feel sick. If the methadone was increased all the medications would work together fine, however, due to the nature of the illnesses many times they would not tell us what medications they were suppose to take. We could not afford to have urine sample screening for everything—shhh… the clients do not know this.

The clients fear being treated differently and often were by various agencies. Unknown to the clients, some of the clinics had begun dosing TB medications just because

TB had again become such a problem. The various county agencies did go to their homes to track patients. Once, we lost one to incarceration because he would not take his TB medications.

Many clients, I believe, need their dose split, half in the morning and half in the evening but this was not possible at our clinic. The concept of a dose increase as the solution never worked for me. I would do anything to prevent an increase simply due to the difficulty in the eventual dose tapering. The fact that many of the clients were driving to and from the clinic and were out on the road, period, was my motivation.

Do not misunderstand me, for many the dose meant stability, not all clients had their abilities impaired. Besides, I come from a holistic point of view. I personally believe the fewer chemicals the better, so the sooner a client could get off methadone the better. However, research has revealed there is more than a seventy-five percent relapse when patients end their methadone treatment.

I am sorry to say, the local hospital was one of the worst offenders of bad treatment. I had been there on several occasions with my parents and later with my clients. I saw the way people were handled if the staff had it in their minds the problem was alcohol or drug related. It was cruel and I no longer wonder why the clients have *attitude*. These people are assigned a label and there is no way society, the agencies, or even they themselves can escape it. I will admit that the cry "I am an addict" was more of an excuse than anything else. I made it very clear to my clients this did not work for me.

I was very lucky, I had a tremendous amount of freedom to practice my style of therapy. I was allowed to pull from my bag-of-tricks whatever I thought would work. Because I handled the worst of the worst abusers—that is not fair, the ones that needed a lot of attention—I continued to get assigned many cases directly from the doctor. I gained the trust of the clinic physician and that meant my job was easier than most.

~ ~ ~

Todd (White Todd) called me down to his office, he was going to assign a client to me which transferred from twenty-one-day detoxification to maintenance. He wanted to tell me about him before I met him. He said this man was a minister who relapsed and blamed it on the stress of a marital separation and not being able to see his children. He had been removed as minister from his congregation with no explanation. The man, after finishing his physical, would be available to see me for a quick session and treatment planning.

As we talked, I understood he was educated and sorrow-filled from missing his wife and children. He also was in a depressed state because of no longer having his congregation. I gave him one of my books on codependency to read. He was living in a shelter and just coming off a drug-run of two weeks. He was not out of my office ten minutes when Todd began asking me what I thought about him. I told him something was wrong with this picture.

About three days later, Todd transfers a phone call to me stating that it was the client's wife and he just transferred her to my caseload. She insisted on treatment and since there was a signed release in her husband's chart she could check on his status. When I answered, the woman began to tell me in a threatening manner that her husband was a child molester, that he had molested their two children, and who knows how many others. She was in the process of pressing charges and she also had a restraining order issued against him. She said that if he did not show up for treatment it was because of his arrest. The call was shocking and in a divorce situation, you just never know.

I did not mention the phone call to Todd, it was more venting than anything else. But there was something about this man I did not like. When he came up for sessions, he talked about adjusting to life and society in general. Even when I needed to confront him with his test results and his continued drug use, he would just want to talk about the kids in the world. He would go into detail about all the children on the street and the moms that pimp them. He told me the last time he was shooting-up he shared a needle with a ten-year-old boy!

I stopped him in mid-sentence, "You are a father, a minister and on the road to recovery but you shared a needle with a ten-year-old boy?"

"Yes," he replied.

"Did you see anything wrong with this?" I asked.

"No." Then he continued saying that the boy had been using, he had been around but did not know where he lived. In his own defense, he said he did not introduce him to the drug but the boy needed some.

I could only remind him of the dangers of sharing needles. I said, "Well, have a nice day and we'll go into this more in our next session."

When he walked out, I was sick. I told myself I would do what I had to do but this was the first client that repulsed me. I never put a hold on his dose or a request to see his counselor again. He was fee detoxed off the program within weeks. I swear I tried not to judge, but it was more than I could handle and still remain nice.

| 5 | The Rules | |

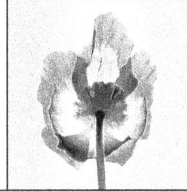

The new intakes were randomly assigned, whoever had the lowest caseload got the next intake duty. One never knew how many intakes there would be in one day. Clients did not have appointments, they were told to show up at 5:30AM and to get in line, first come first served. The procedure was simple, the client had to demonstrate that he had an addiction, prior treatment, or prior treatment failure. If a client had MediCal, it had to be active, if not it was two hundred dollars per month. For the twenty-one-day detox, half of the fee was due upfront, and twelve dollars per day thereafter.

Computer systems were linked up so a counselor could contact all the methadone clinics within three hundred miles to check for double dosing, see where the client came from, and get all their records. Very few people had never been on the program, or at least not tried the twenty-one-day detox. I might as well say it: I believe that the twenty-one-day detoxification program for anyone was a setup for failure, despite the client's optimism. Withdrawal from heroin usually takes seven days; withdrawal from methadone, depending on how long it has been taken, can last up to thirty days. The worst part of most programs is when the methadone treatment phase is over, so is the counseling—just when it is needed the most!

Intakes needed to present a urine sample, a blood test, a TB test, and a complete general physical; for women, this included pregnancy screening. A client coming off a drug-run usually had several other problems to address; malnutrition, infection, diabetes, hypertension, heart disease, bronchitis, emphysema, epilepsy, liver disease, asthma, poor oral hygiene and tooth decay, and this is not even beginning to address all the psychological factors or family issues.

My initial thoughts were how do you address all of this in fifteen minutes every two weeks? The real problem was to get the fifteen minutes without holding their dose which always turned in to a good conversation blocker. They could and would rant for weeks on how you once ruined their entire life with only one held dose.

The only way you could find out their medical history was to hold their hand and walk them to the doctor, so I did this on many occasions. Again, on behalf of the clients, I could not blame them for the attitude. Despite the consequence of their being stuck at a methadone clinic most likely for life, I saw and heard of many abuses.

Drug and alcohol counseling is a fairly new job classification. Most licensed professionals will not work with this population and little consideration for therapy was being given in prior years, far less expecting a positive treatment outcome. It was sad, yet almost humorous to watch the logic a counselor used to analyze clients and the methodology utilized in the clinic. Mine included part commonsense, part parenting skills, a little dog training, some of what I learned in school, lots of humor, sincere concern and consideration; but most of all, instinct. Many of my clients felt heard and listened to for the first time. I had to calibrate my survival skills too. I could make my life hard, their life hard, or I could find the middle ground where everyone gets what they want or need.

~ ~ ~

Back to my first day of testing, I had gone through most of my caseload by 9:30AM and I was still intact. I had my sense of humor and everything was completed the way it was supposed to be. I looked at the clock and was grateful that there was only five minutes until lunch. Despite everything, I was actually hungry!

The area was neat and tidy. I was at attention awaiting the next client when the loudspeaker barked out I had a call on line one. It was another counselor at our clinic.

"Allie?" she asked.

"Yes," I responded.

"One of Jane's babies died and that is all I have to say," she reported calmly.

The counselor hung-up. You could have hit me with a truck at a hundred miles per hour and I would have felt better. Jane was my first client, the one who had her children taken from her. Just then a client came up and said, "You're my new counselor and you're testing today."

I was in a fog but managed, "Yes, your name?"

He performed, returned the sample and I think I said thank you and cleared the dose. Later that day, someone asked me to lock the doors and I did. Then I ran upstairs and found the counselor who left me hanging with Jane.

"Please, you must tell me more," I begged.

Aretha was a quiet woman who kept to herself. She suffered from obesity. Once she sat in her chair, she did not get up except to get her food. She had several physical ailments, mostly due to her weight. The clients trusted her due to her confidentiality code, it was also rumored she had been married to a heroin addict once. The clinic always had lots of gossip; it was hard not to hear the most recent rumor. Besides, we all learned what was up with each other because somehow all was shared to someone at some time. The clinic had very few secrets.

Aretha was always eating, it started at 5:30AM and probably never stopped. She was a good person, do not misunderstand me, but not unlike most of the counselors, she had her issues too. As she was organizing her lunch she began with, "I most likely shouldn't tell you this but what the hell, it will hit the newspaper tomorrow."

And it did just that! Have you ever had to hold back an emotion? I mean something that is gut-wrenching, jerk your heart out, ringing in your ears kind of emotion? An emotion where you can hear your heartbeat in your head and beads of sweat form on your face? I had a lump in my throat and tears beginning to form. I wanted, and now needed, more information. Jane on a drug-run? It seemed obvious since ditching me for the one appointment; the temper tantrum on Friday; not showing over the weekend; and, she had yet to show up today. I needed more facts!

As Aretha shook the salt on her lunch I said, "What the hell do you mean her kid died and that's all you have to say? Talk to me!"

Aretha began, "You know I never could stand that bitch, Jane. She never came up for sessions, was a real problem with testing, and all I felt that she ever cared about was crack."

"Yes," I said, "go on."

"The woman who got custody of Jane's two kids is on my caseload," she continued.

"You mean her comrade?"

"Yeah," she answered as she cut a piece of meat and put it in her mouth.

I said, "Go on."

"Well, she was arrested this morning for the death of the three-year-old and the infant was taken into Foster Care due to all of the cigarette burns and the burn from the iron on its thigh."

I meekly said, "What?"

"You heard me and I ain't gonna say anymore," she replied without missing a chew.

I got up and as I walked away said, "Thank you." I did not know what I feared the most, if Jane showed up after lunch for her session, or if she did not.

I felt physically ill, common I guess when you try to deny emotions. Most of my caseload had come in for testing and the whispers of the rumor-mill had already started: "You are Jane's counselor aren't you?" "Did you hear?" "Have you seen Jane?"

Then Jane came in, sorry, but it was an awkward performance for the drama queen. No words of "Ahhh, my son died," but instead, "Ahhh, I need take-homes."

So ended some of the illusion, but my education and disconnection began. I knew Jane was hurting, I could see it in her eyes, I could feel it. I could also sense her current *game*. To top-it-off, she accused me of having the nerve to demand a urine test from her on the day of the murder of her son. *Oh well*, I thought to myself.

It was common when someone died who was connected to the clinic to have a carwash to raise funds for the funeral. Our Director allowed posters to be displayed. So the next day, Jane showed up with the carwash posters and her take-home box. She looked better than I had ever seen her. Then she brought up the issue of her MediCal and the almighty dose.

"Well, do I lose it if my son dies or do I get Social Security?" she asked. She knew better than me that her MediCal would quickly be taken away because the children had been removed from her custody.

Jane continued on her crack-run, her MediCal was soon terminated due to the loss of her children, and she went into fee detox. She came around a couple of times after that but the local girls had gotten it into their heads that Jane was responsible for the abuse of the infant and no one takes to child abusers. If Jane was around, something of a riot ensued. Eventually, she became a fourteen-day no show. By the way, it was also rumored that Jane stole all the money for the funeral that was collected at the carwash.

~ ~ ~

When I first started, Todd (Black Todd) was responsible for doing all the intakes of the clients coming onto the program. Todd claimed to have been raised by heroin addicts back East and was a born-again Christian. He had been able to right his ways through the power of Jesus Christ which was great for him but some of the clients grew weary and complained of his overzealous manner. When the rules changed, the clients had their initial clinical assessment done by their assigned counselor. This put Todd solely responsible for chart reviews, which unless you had food to feed him, could be brutal. Call it a bribe, call it survival, but I made my life easier by always having food ready for Black Todd.

Black Todd was memorable not just because he ate nonstop, but by *what* he ate. He could not get it spicy enough and when he "got down" on one of the local burritos, we would watch his head and face break out in a sweat for half an hour. Again, it was the little things that kept our day interesting, "Let's watch Toddy eat!"

Often, the initial clinical assessment was the time when you could establish a relationship with the client. If it was a good experience, it was a good relationship. Awareness was the key. A client is in a stage of withdrawal at the time of intake. The best description I can give is to try to imagine the worst case of the stomach flu or food poisoning you have ever had; your head is pounding, there is nausea and/or imminent diarrhea, aching bones, cold sweats—you know, just plain miserable.

The client while feeling these symptoms has to find a way to the clinic before 5:30AM with no guarantee of treatment and no idea how long it would take. They were forced to being interviewed for an hour, observed urinating, give blood usually with no available veins and many time a sincere fear of needles, and given a full physical examination. This was all done generally with no consideration for their present physical or mental state of being. Truly a hurry-up-and-wait procedure. A little consideration and a few kind words went a long way; I used this time to be the nice guy.

Most of the clients have been on the program before so it did not take me long to learn that the information I needed was already in the files. When I was told of the name of the intake, I pulled the discharge file and confirmed the information or any changes. It was very hard to get more than a nod with a person ready to puke any second. I formulated a minimal treatment plan which could be modified at any time, and it usually did need changing as soon as the physical and lab reports came back.

I also gave them "Allie's Rules" and made sure even if nothing else was clear, these rules were to be remembered. I had them repeat the list to me:

1. Do not ever piss-off the lady at the window. She is the one who controls the money and you may need to ask her for a favor someday.
2. Always be kind, polite, and do not ever piss-off the dispensing nurses, they can make your future hell.
3. Do not ever piss-off the doctor or curse within his hearing space, everything must be approved by him.
4. Keep a low profile, get your dose, and get out of here.
5. I will treat you with respect and I expect it in return. I am the only one here that is paid to be your friend. The luckiest day you ever had

is today, getting me for your counselor. Do not ever forget this.

6. You get one chance, I will not put a hold on your dose as long as you always come to see me when the nurse tells you to see your counselor. One chance, that is it.

With these rules, my clients learned to respect that sometimes the line was long due to the time of day, urine testing, or if there was a need to change the bottle. There could be a delay or doctors orders may call for delays, there was always those possibilities. My clients knew they could wait in line for twenty minutes to get to the window and the nurse may tell them there was a hold on their dose. This could be upsetting to anyone but our clients did not have the right to be upset or complain about anything.

One day, I was sitting in my office looking out the window to see which client I would approach next, when I heard my name called to the dispensing area immediately for a *chunk check*. When I arrived at the area, there were two other counselors, including Jack, in the dispensing room with Moses. They were all laughing at me.

"What part of this duty do you not understand?" Jack asked in his sarcastic tone. "If your client throws-up his dose and comes back for more, you must go look at his chunks, *vomit* to be polite. You need to verify that the methadone came up before a second dose can be given."

"Get out of here," I squirmed thinking he must be kidding.

"It's the law," said the nurse.

If there is one thing I cannot handle, it is vomit. I never allowed my daughters to do it; one daughter did it once but she made it to the toilet. *Mind power* I told them and it worked! Even today, just the sounds of gagging can make me hurl.

So my client who was standing at the front door holding his stomach said, "I'm sorry, it's over here."

I walked to the planter, I saw something pink and started to gag. I returned, obviously looking quite sick, and told the nurse, "Give it to him."

They were only given half of the initial dose if they threw up the first. After that, I added a new rule to my list:

7. Do not ever, ever vomit at the clinic.

The staff had a good laugh but *none* of my clients ever got sick at the clinic again.

6 | Supporting Eleanor

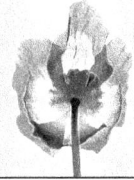

The doctor called me down to his office and requested a client's chart. I had just been assigned the client and had not yet met with her. At one time, we were allowed to wait two weeks for an assessment, but that did not last long. The new client transferred to the program from another clinic, this was her first time here. The doctor wanted to see if they had done a pregnancy test on her. He pointed out that within the three days on the program at our clinic her stomach had bloated, he wanted to rule out pregnancy. The chart indicated the test had been performed but results were not back yet. We had pregnancy kits which showed results immediately but they were rarely utilized.

The doctor peered through the dosing window and stated she was in line and to see if I could grab her. I quickly got to the dosing window just as she swallowed her dose. She agreed to meet with me in one of the nearby examining rooms. We were not supposed to do this, but I got to do some things others did not because of my relationship with the doctor. Doing this was very awkward, like *hello, I have never met you before but you appear to have gained twenty pounds in the last three days, when was your last period?* Somehow, I managed to pull it off. Eleanor was a really cool person. I wish in so many ways we had talked about her life experiences more than actual counseling, I am sure she had a very interesting story. Of course, there was not one person who I had met at the clinic that did not have at least one good jaw-dropping tale to share.

Eleanor laughed hard when I got around to the big question. She said, "Hell no, I am not pregnant. I got my tubes tied after my second child, I couldn't see bringing in anymore children like some people do, considering you know… Besides, I haven't had sex in years, not that I wouldn't like to."

She told me that she had not been feeling well and moved to be closer to a clinic because she had a hard time getting around, she had never gotten her driver's license. She lived a block or two from the clinic now. I suggested that she make an appointment with the doctor across the street and she agreed stating she was pretty sure what the problem was, "It's my liver." This happened before we had the facts on Hepatitis C.

I asked her why she thought she had a liver problem. She explained that her mother had just died of cirrhosis and she had two uncles who died of it. She was still mourning the loss of her mother. She had two daughters, nine and eleven years of age, and three sisters who lived upstairs in her house.

Eleanor had been some sort of female gang leader at one time and had all the scars to prove it. She knew everyone at the clinic and with her approval of me as a counselor, I had entered one more corner of acceptance in the culture. After our meeting, I walked with her to the doctor's office across the street and assisted her with the appointment to see Dr. Chan. When I returned, I shared the information with our clinic doctor.

Sadly, he confirmed Eleanor's self-diagnosis, "I thought so. Good job Allie."

~ ~ ~

I walked by Javier's office and a client was hanging all over him, "Ahh, cm'on Javier, lemme on the prooogram," she crooned.

"Susan, get off me," he said.

"Don't you like me anymore Javier?"

"Yes, of course I like you Susan. I am trying to get some work done. Hey, Allie, have you met Susan yet?" he asked as he spied me.

"No, Javier, I don't think I have," I replied with a smile.

"Oh, Hiiiiii Allieeeeeee, what do yooooooo do here? She is pretty Javier. Are you a counselor? Pleaseeee tell himmm to let me on the program today. Pleasssseeee be my counselor, pleaseeeeeeee. Look at this," Susan said as she started to remove her blouse to reveal the abscess on her right breast. "Seeee, I neeeeed medical attention."

"Susan, put your shirt on and get out of here. Go sit in the lobby and I will ask the doctor and Allie if you can get on the program today. You should have been here this morning," Javier scowled at her.

"I know Javier but I couldn't get a ride. I am here now, pleasseeee Javier."

"Go sit in the lobby," he instructed.

"Okay, but you hurt my feelings," she glanced downward.

As Susan left the room, Javier rolled his eyes, "She is something else!"

"I guess so," I said in return. I learned quickly that there was no such thing as modesty at the clinic, as well as, political correctness.

Javier asked, "Would you mind taking her on? She has been with all the other counselors and she already likes you."

I said, "Sure, I don't care." Javier asked me to go inquire if Doc would mind doing a late intake. I went to the doctor and he knew already what I was about to ask him.

He said, "What difference does it make, she'll leave the program soon. We should only take people who really want to work the program. Well, bring her back and get her chart from the last time she was here."

I passed her in the lobby, she was different somehow than most of the clients. When I walked by, she grabbed me, gave me a big hug and asked again, "Pleasssseeeeeee be my counselor." She was like a child, I could not tell if she were seriously mentally retarded, brain damaged, or on drugs. She may have been high but then again, maybe not.

Susan was a challenge, it was more like babysitting than counseling. She did not belong on this program, or the street, she was not like the rest. She had just given birth to twins, her third set I discovered, not to mention her other two children. This girl had delivered eight children and she was a child herself! She was twenty-three years old and out of the hospital from delivering her twins just one day. Mind you, I also got to see the stitches from her delivery, it was a Cesarean thank God. Knowing Susan, she would have shown me her episiotomy if she had had one!

We got Susan on the program that day, she stated she needed lots and lots of counseling. I told her I would see her whenever she needed to talk. She was so full of love, and again, so childlike. She reappeared the next day just before 10:00AM. She came up to my office and began to tell her story. I did not know what to think, we would talk but it was like talking to a child. She continued to arrive at the clinic just before lunch and would sit there for at least an hour. Sometimes she would bring her lunch to eat while we talked. I really thought she just had nowhere to go and needed the attention.

Susan told me she had a strange childhood with many different fathers. She had dropped out of school in the seventh grade because she knew she was different. Her mother had kept Susan's first child and one set of twins. The other children had been adopted by members of her mother's church. The two children she delivered the week before were premature and still in the hospital. It was so difficult to piece this story together, like trying to get information from a seven-year-old with Attention Deficit Disorder.

She was basically homeless. She and her "husband" had a hotel room but usually slept in his van. It was a different sort of marriage, she did not always stay with him. We talked about drugs; I discovered that her husband was smoking crack. I suggested this was not a good thing and stated he should stop. The next day, she brought me his crack pipe and some crack!

Now I panicked and thought *What the hell do I do with this stuff?* We flushed the drugs down the toilet and tossed the pipe in the trash. The next day when she showed up with a black eye, it was no surprise. What *was* surprising was her response; she said it was no big deal, she was used to it.

I asked Susan about social workers, she could not remember. I asked her about Welfare, she did not know. Her mother handled it all and is refusing to talk to her right now. I was beyond frustrated. I spoke to the doctor, I spoke to Javier; there was nothing we could do and it was obvious, they did not appear to care. She may have needed methadone for her addiction but she did not appear to be able to care for herself. Then again, she survived on the streets, something I could never do.

Susan talked about the babies like she might get custody which really scared me so I asked permission to call her mother, to try to get some sort of concrete information. Her mother turned out to be similar to an acquaintance of mine. They had lived the wild life in their youth and the effects on the children did not surface until school authorities got involved, or Social Services. The parents found a path to live sober but the children had remained wild . Now, it was like trying to break a wild horse. If the children did not follow the teachings of the newly found religion, they would be locked-out of the house. Susan simply stated that the Bible study was boring and she could not sit still that long.

Susan's mother was polite but could not take the drama anymore. She had three of the children and was helping with the other's adoptions. If Susan could follow the rules, she was welcome to come home but she had gone through enough heartbreak. I was powerless. The only other thing I could do was to report her as a danger to herself and others. This might have cost me my job, besides, I was not quite sure she was a danger to others.

Susan eventually lost her temporary MediCal due to the loss of custody of her children. She was put on fee detox and was back on the street. She came around a couple of times for condoms and was high on drugs, I never saw her again. This client taught me how easy it was to cross the emotional involvement line. Some things I just had no control over, some people just fell through the cracks in the system.

~ ~ ~

Eleanor called me from home and asked if I could see her when she got her dose. Within ten minutes, she was at the clinic. She called me from the lobby stating that she could not walk up the stairs and could I please meet with her downstairs. Only two weeks had passed and her abdomen appeared to be larger than before. She had a bag full of prescriptions to be cleared. She did indeed have Hepatitis C and the cirrhosis was beyond repair. She was trying to be optimistic but our doctor stated that if she lived more than six months it would be a miracle.

Eleanor needed help, she was trying to get better but she only knew what she only knew, she was sick. She was surrounded by people that did not necessarily have evil intentions but certainly did not know how to adequately care for her or supervise her children in a proper manner, whatever *proper manner* means. I was uncomfortable with her prescriptions. She had Valium, codeine, and diuretics, as well as, the methadone which we were to begin tapering immediately. Thank God alcohol was not an issue.

This was a complicated case. Here at the clinic, we were trying to get less of everything going through her liver, while other doctors gave her more. She needed to be on a strict diet; she had several medical appointments to get to; and, she needed to take her medication on time. She had a charming s/o (significant other) but he was not clean, he was on and off the program due to the cost and his lack of commitment to being clean. By the way, *clean* means not actively using drugs. I later found out Eleanor's sisters were not clean either.

Most of our sessions, and there were a lot of them, were about her children. Again, she was trying to do the right things. I helped her get the school uniforms and the tutoring she could not afford for her kids. Transportation was an issue for her and there were times I would drive her to the hospital for her tests. I did these things on my way home or on my lunch hour, all close by the clinic. I had given her applications for a transportation service but they never made it to the agency.

As Eleanor's health worsened, so did her family affairs. She was losing her oldest daughter to the streets and felt powerless. After only three months, Eleanor was in a wheelchair and the family was more harmful than helpful. She could not make sure the girls got to school each day and really could not depend on anyone else. It was not the younger ones she worried about so much, but the oldest girls who gave her the most difficulty. A very stupid incident happened at school due to the time and recent changes in the school district's approach, she was expelled.

It truly made me wonder; here we had a kid, not bad but on the edge, and the only structure she had was now removed. The school district allowed her to participate in homestudy with a teacher who would come by the house once a week to check on her progress. What would the other choice be, Foster Care? Within months, Eleanor's worst fears came true, the child was having sex and using drugs. After a few weeks the child had her first run-in with the police, this sent Eleanor on her first trip to the hospital.

Eleanor was one of the people who I had met at the program that was deathly afraid needles. Often, women get involved with drugs through their men, s/o. The men would do the injecting for them if needed. The thing that made it so bad was after years of intravenous drug use it is difficult, if not impossible, to find a vein or an artery. One day, Dr. Chan called me and asked if I would go to the hospital and calm Eleanor down while she received her medication. We talked about her case. He told me that often when a patient was taken to the hospital with liver disease and the drainage was started, it was not long before the liver would just give out completely. Evidently, the body cannot handle the draining process more than a few times.

Eleanor was scared and I was most likely the only sober person she knew. The IV drip was in her neck, the only vein they could use and they had a hard time with that one. We kept the focus positive and created a plan of action for her oldest daughter. She kept sharing her dreams with me about her mother, Mother's Day was always hard for her.

Eleanor had made it past the six-month mark and our clinic doctor was amazed. However, she was in more pain and needed to take a simple prescription four times daily or she would appear to be drunk; she would not be able to think clearly, or speak clearly. Apparently, the disease causes a buildup of toxins in the blood. I believe she needed to be in an assisted living facility, just my opinion.

7 Gays, Needles, and HIV

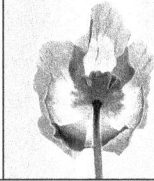

As I walked into the dispensing area it all looked like a typical Tuesday morning, the clients in line, the reception area filled. I placed my chart in the box for the doctor's review. As usual, only 8:30AM and the building was full. Hangovers from Monday's dose changes?

I heard a woman's loud voice which I did not recognize. "That's her, I want her, the one with the nice ass."

"Chill Rita," I said, "you can't talk like that, behave yourself."

"Allie, how many do you have on your caseload?" she asked.

"I don't know, what difference does it make?"

"You have a point, can I talk to you?"

"Sure, step into my private office," I said as we went into the urine observation room for our private, well, not even close to private chat. I was stuck no matter what I heard now. I already gave it away that she could be assigned to me. I could say yes, despite the story; or, I could be in for an unknown future revenge, and say no.

I got a little of the story from her. She was a long-timer, just got released from prison, and her partner (girlfriend) was getting on the program. As I investigated the case, I was told this client was *trouble-based*; and of course, I was most likely the one who could handle her. I was the only one that had not been assigned to her at one time or another.

It was like "old home week" at the clinic. All the program clients would say "Hi" to the just released ones. I saw and heard Eleanor tell the new girl, "Hey, homegirl, when did you get out?" Then she turned to face me, "Hey Allie, I did time with this bitch, she is good people." Turning again to Rita, "Hey, try to get my counselor."

"She did and I am," I told Eleanor.

Rita looked at me and said, "You're cute."

"Get your hands off my counselor, she is not that way," Eleanor quickly told her.

"How do you know?" Rita said. They both cracked-up laughing.

"Good to see you but I got to get my dose and get out of here," Eleanor told Rita. "Come by sometime, counselor knows where I live. Give her directions, Allie" and she rolled off in her wheelchair.

Rita asked, "Hey, what's up with my homegirl?"

"Later, you know we can't discuss those things," I said.

"Oh shit, you're one of *those* counselors."

"We will talk later when I don't have an audience," I said. All the counselors and the Director had gathered to watch the group disperse. I inquired if the paperwork was complete and it was but she had yet to see the doctor. I advised Ethel at the front desk to let the doctor know I was interviewing the client.

This was another thing I did to help them feel comfortable. Why make them sit there? So I said, "Come on, you want a cup of coffee?"

Rita got a serious look on her face as she wondered what I was up to, being so nice and all. "That would be great," she finally responded.

So we got our coffee which was more like a cup of sugar liquefied with milk and a drop of coffee for color effect. This was the way most of the clients drank their coffee. I gave her my spiel; low profile, respect for respect, and just do not lie to me, and so on.

She looked up and said, "You're different, you ever use?"

"No," I said with a smile and added, "I am educated."

She laughed then said, "Serious, how did a classy broad like you end up here?"

I laughed at her and said, "What can't you believe? This was a career choice." I told her my story and my philosophy about addiction.

"I am gonna like you," she said.

Just then the doctor called my office for Rita and we went down for the physical examination. The doctor started in with, "Oh, Rita what are we to do with you? You were clean when you got out, what happened?"

"Oh, you know Doc, I am an addict. What else is an addict to do? So you need me to piss Doc? I gotta go now."

"Sure Rita, go. Allie, you take her."

"Okay," I said and took Rita to get her specimen. I told her to get in touch with me after the physical so she could sign the treatment plan. Then she could get her dose and was out of here. She gave me a thumbs-up and walked back to the medical examination rooms.

I walked directly into the reception area and sat myself next to Rita's girlfriend and said, "Your Rita is something else."

The beautiful auburn haired, hazel-eyed woman looked up with a big smile and said, "Yes she is. My name is Katy and you are Allie?"

"Yes, glad to meet you," I extended my hand.

She took it and shook it in a businesslike manner. I inquired if she were getting on the program and she said that she did not have enough money. She had lost her MediCal and would need to wait until next week.

I said bluntly, "You know this won't work if you are using."

She said, "I know, we are prepared. We only have enough stuff for me and we promised each other that we were not going to buy any more, we are making plans to move. We've got to get out of this town if we are going to get it together."

"That sounds like a smart move. How long do you think it will take to get it together?" I asked.

She said, "We hope to get going soon."

However, their plan was doomed to failure. Just when I started to get excited about goal oriented behavior too. But I said, "Hey, that's great, when you see Rita tell her to come to my office upstairs, it was nice meeting you Katy."

I walked back to my office thinking about the family dynamics with an invalid mother, a teenage boy, a daughter that shows up once in a while, two grandchildren two and four years old, and Katy and Rita—the all-American family.

A bit later, Rita came running in fearful of a long lecture which she was sure would come. "Hey, I'll get Katy on the program right away and I am not going to use, don't worry."

"That is the last thing I worry about," I said. "Just don't lie and let me know how I can help."

"You can get me my dose and let me get out of here," Rita stated matter-of-factly.

I said, "Sign here and it's a deal. Oh, by the way, are you going to get a job?"

She laughed as she walked out the door, turned and said, "Right."

I quickly learned three things about Rita; she drove like a maniac, she would come every day just before closing, and she was *dirty*. Well, we were supposed to language this in a more positive way—she was actively using illegal substances. Rita also had a quick, bad temper, she was a fighter.

Just as they say, nobody likes a child abuser. Well, even in this crowd it was not handled well, and the word was out about the death of Jane's son. Rita had other agenda's with Jane, she was out to get her. She even questioned me and how I could be Jane's counselor. Word traveled fast and the rumor was there was a *hit* out on Jane, just as in the movies. When I got the warning, I just sat there thinking to myself *How did I end up with these two on my caseload and how in hell do I deal with this?* [Note: This was not the last time I asked myself this question.]

One time, there was a slight confrontation between these two in the dispensing line. This was the first time I actually heard directly from the doctor and the Director at the same time, "Allie, get control of your clients." I used the power of methadone dosing, be good clients or no dose. For a week, I asked them both to come at different times. That worked until Jane disappeared.

Then all the sessions with Rita surrounded mothers, motherhood, and how all these women at the clinic took good care of their children. Finally, the question came, "What do you think happened to Jane?"

I got the phone call, Jane had died.

~ ~ ~

Jane, my first client. Some we take in harder than others, we just did not talk about it. Again, I experienced suppressed emotions. I could not get any more information and what made it worse was I had her brother on my caseload. He and I had not talked much about his sister other than he thought she was the female version of Satan and had been since birth. He, in my opinion, could not possibly be related to her. He was clean cut, working, and clean. He was working the program the way it was designed to work and only came once a week.

Most of the counselors put up some sort of "In memory of..."note on the bulletin board. I was asked to write something also. I was uncomfortable about doing this because I did not have much information about her, but I wrote a poem in her memory.

> Today I heard my first client died.
> On my way home all I could do was cry.
> Why couldn't I find the right words to say
> To somehow help her find her way?
> Alone, confused, hurt, and lost
> She drugged her pain, not caring of cost.
> Next time you tell me you made a mistake
> Together we'll look at photos of the last wake.
> You and I know it is Russian roulette
> Who will be next, should we make a bet?

It's hard to maintain this level of care
While our hearts go through this wear and tear.
May Jane's soul finally rest in peace
Joining in spirit with her son
Please God, at least.

The Director asked me to put the poem up with a photo of Jane. I told him I was uncomfortable because in my gut I did not think she was dead, do not ask me why. I asked if it could wait until I talked to her brother.

Javier agreed, "Hey that's a good idea. I got it Allie, don't put that up until you see her brother."

Jane's brother came in the next morning, produced a urine sample and was in a great mood. When I asked him if he could please come up to my office, he said he was in a hurry and asked if it could wait. I told him it was kind of important and I needed to do this in my office. As much as it was discouraged and as much as it was questionable, we did lots of counseling sessions in the parking lot, but not this time.

He walked in and sat down, I offered coffee and made sure the tissue box was handy. I do not think he had a clue of what I was about to ask him. I did not want to be the one to tell him but I guess it was better than Rita shouting something across the parking lot.

I began with, "We don't talk about this, but you know I was your sister Jane's counselor?"

"Yeah, what did she do now?" he asked.

"Well, I heard a couple of days ago, well, that she died due to an overdose," I stumbled.

"What?" he said, "Wishful thinking. You know, I couldn't bring myself to go to her baby's funeral?"

"So you don't think she is dead?" I asked meekly.

"No, I think the family would have celebrated. Can I use your phone? I'll call my other sister Ruby." No one answered. "I am sure the family would be looking for money for a funeral. I am sure she is still out there."

"Well, the Director wants to put this up," I said as I handed him the poem. "I thought we should talk to you first. I hope you don't mind."

He glanced at the writing and said, "That is nice but she is still alive, I'm sure."

Three months later, I had a call on the intercom. I picked up the phone, "This is Allie, can I help you?"

"Allie? My counselor Allie?"

"Who is this?" I asked.

"This is Jane. I just wanted to say hello and let you know that I was doing good."

"Jane! Where are you? It was rumored you were dead. Everyone thought you were dead!" I shrieked.

"Yeah, my brother told me. He also said you were the only person who ever said anything nice about me and that I should call you. I just wanted to let you know that I am in a Christian Home and have turned my life over to Christ. I have been clean for two months."

"Hey, that's great Jane, keep up the good work," I smiled to myself.

She said, "God bless."

That was the last I heard from Jane. The rules were changed after this, we no longer put up little "In memory of…" posters.

~ ~ ~

Daniel, Jane's brother, had been assigned to me just before Jane had disappeared. We were doing the intake when he mentioned that he had a sister that used to be on the program but not to confuse the two of them being anything alike. This previous conversation and my inquiring of Jane's death was the only time we spoke of her. Daniel was good-looking and had all his teeth with a smile you knew got him into trouble. He told me he had been clean for years and did not know why he started using but he did not want to go down the same road he had before. So he was getting on the program to get clean and to stay clean.

Just separating from his wife of fifteen years, Daniel had three children ages fifteen, nine, and two. He said his wife threw him out because of the drug use and as much as he missed them there was no hope for reconciliation. I figured we would talk about this issue later. He was articulate and motivated. I rarely had the chance to make up a true treatment plan and have someone work it, Daniel wanted to try. He needed and wanted take-homes fast. He already had a job, a real job with a paycheck stub and taxes paid. He had to pay cash for his treatment and it was a financial strain. I was able to do my job with Daniel and it was working well. He utilized his sessions, in fact, I saw Daniel every week. He was on a scheduled taper of his dose and all seemed very optimistic.

When Daniel was in the third month of treatment, he called to make an appointment to speak with me the next day. I asked if it was anything I could help with now and he said he was leaving his doctor's office, they had let him use the phone there. He would see me at 5:30AM the next morning and he wanted cream, no sugar in his coffee. After I had spent enough time doing the *"I wonder what…"* game in my mind, I found his chart and looked through it for a clue. I soon put the chart away for the night and went home.

Daniel's car was in the lot when I pulled up at 5:15AM. I invited him up to my office and we had small talk while the coffee was brewing. We took the coffee into my office then he began, "Almost everything I have told you is a lie."

My first thought was that he was a DEA agent spying on the clinic. So I said, "Okay, you are a DEA agent. I don't think I have broken the rules, can I take the Fifth?"

He laughed then asked, "I hear that if you have HIV you get methadone for free."

"That is true," I told him, "there is a grant program through the Ryan White Foundation where treatment, including many other services, are free."

"I'm HIV positive," he stated with his head down. "I didn't tell anyone before because I was ashamed. That is the real reason I left my family, they don't even know. I can't afford the methadone anymore and my doctor told me I might be able to get it for free here. If I can't, he knows of a clinic that does have it free, but I don't want to lose you as my counselor."

Numb with emotion, I put my shrink-hat on and said, "You know I will get you free treatment, the most important thing right now is what your secret has cost you. Do you think this is fair to your wife?"

"Do you think this is fair to me?" he responded.

"It was your choice to use a dirty needle," I told him.

He was my first HIV positive patient and like most, he remembered the moment he contracted the disease. As with an unwanted pregnancy, most women can tell you the minute they got pregnant. He said he had been clean for years when he and his wife bought a house. They were just starting to get ahead when she told him she was pregnant with their two-year-old.

"I should have been happy but I was pissed," he continued. "I told her I didn't want any more kids, we had a fight. I left, and of course, the worst of my homeboys were there waiting for me. I had a 'I don't give a damn' attitude and used. I swear I only used that one time. I went home, we kissed and made-up. The baby came and life was doing okay. Then I got this job and they made me take a physical, that is when I found out I was positive. I went out and used again. Then I used the drugs as an excuse to get thrown-out of the house." He took a long deep breath.

I asked if he had brought anything from his doctor or a list of his medications. He had everything with him. I called Ethel and asked if we had any Ryan White slots available and she said, "Yes, for who?"

I said I would take care of that later with her but to hold the slot for me. She said no problem and I turned to Daniel, "There you go. Let me make copies of the papers and you can be on your way."

When I returned, I suggested he get into a group regarding this issue. He said he had tried one but they were mostly for gays and he could not relate. I later discovered, this was pervasive. HIV-positive heterosexuals had very few support groups in the immediate proximity.

I told Daniel, "Thank you for your trust, we'll talk more about this later."

We shared a hug and he was off to work. He had forgotten to dose and I forgot to remind him. I had all the paperwork in order for his free treatment.

The rest of the day, I was in a fog. I went to Susie's office and to see the doctor for as much information as I could get about HIV. I needed to know Daniel's T-cell count so I knew where we were, no one was checking the viral load yet. Susie did not know of any good groups to send him to either. The end of the day came and I did not want to go home, I stopped by the mall to wander around. I found a store selling bracelets with a percentage of the cost going to AIDS research, I bought one. I still wear the bracelet to this day in memory of my first positive client and the others with the disease.

Daniel continued to do well for a few months. We had to up his dose due to his medication interaction, at least that is what he told me. The truth was he had started drinking. One day he missed, a no show. I had to take away one of his take-homes. About three weeks later, he told me he had to go to court for a DUI. He had not been coming up to talk as much and I left him alone.

I had managed to develop "the look" as a counselor. You know *that* look, an understanding without words. The rest of my clients, as well as, Daniel knew that I knew when they were doing things they should not be doing. I could tell and I called them on it, no urine sample needed. Daniel soon became a fourteen day no show. I did not hear from him for several months, then one day a phone call, "Allie, you have a call on line three."

"Hello, my name is Susana Jones. I know you have rules and cannot give me any information but I have a client on my caseload who says he is a friend of yours and wondered if you could help him."

I asked, "What is your friend's name?"

"We could both get into trouble but please understand that I am trying to do a good thing here. Can I call you at home tonight?" the stranger asked.

"Sure," I said and gave her my phone number. She called me at home that evening. When the phone rang, I figured it was for one of the girls completely forgetting the phone call during work. Then my daughter shouts, "Mom, it's a Susana for you."

I got on the phone and she said, "Hello Allie, yes, his name is Daniel, you were his counselor."

Susana went on to tell me that Daniel was on her caseload because he is HIV positive and he was in jail. She was trying to get him in some sort of program and he was very depressed, she was worried about him.

"What can I do?" I asked.

She said, "If you could write a letter regarding how he behaved in treatment with you, that would help. But more than anything, he needs a friend to write to."

I gave her the address of the clinic and told her Daniel could write me there. I wrote him twice, then he was transferred. I did not get the new address and I never received another letter.

8 Linda's Attempt to Change the System

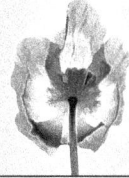

I had my first run-in of many with Javier. He came to my office at 1:15PM, I was finishing up a case note and he requested a chart on one of my clients. I located the chart and gave it to him. He opened it and shrieked, "Where in hell is the annual review for this client?"

"The what?" I asked unknowingly.

"The annual review, you have not done it have you?" he said in an accusing tone.

"No," I said meekly.

"I don't give a damn what the hell you have to do, this better be completed today," he stated emphatically.

He shrieked a few other things relating to the importance of the document and how could I possibly be so completely incompetent. He left me in tears. I did not have a clue, the clients requiring the annual reviews came *from* Javier the month before they were due. The counselor who had the client previously should have completed the document before I even received the chart. I was clueless as what to do.

The document had to be signed by the client, the counselor, the chart reviewer, and the doctor and it was a time sensitive document. I would never backdate a document and there was no way I would forge a client's signature. I was shaking. *Was this a test of my integrity and what I would do to get the job done?*

Looking at the chart, I knew I had met with this person, she and her husband were on the program. I fell in love with their daughter. They seemed to be nice people. Being the totally unreasonable person that I am, I actually tried the phone number listed for the client. I asked the person who answered the phone, "Is Mona there?"

"No, she isn't but I can get a message to her, is this important?"

"Well, yes, this is a friend of hers, my name is Allie. I'll be at this number for a few more minutes."

Mona had been on the program for years and much to my surprise called me back immediately. I was downstairs talking to Black Todd, he noticed I was upset and inquired why. I told him the story and he said not to mention that he talked to me, but not to worry about it. If I got the client to sign the review sometime this week, it would be okay. He said Javier discovered that several annual reviews had not been completed and mine must have been the final blow, he had just lost it. Normally, he said Javier was not like this and please not to quit. He told me not to expect my client to call back. The phone rang.

Mona thought it was time for the annual review and invited me to come over to her house. She would offer to come down to the clinic right away but she did not have a ride. I told her that Todd had just explained if she signed the paper tomorrow, I would be allowed to live. She laughed and said she would see me tomorrow morning. Like I thought, a nice person. As I hung-up the phone, Javier came over to me. He began to apologize for his behavior. I told him I had just gotten off the phone with the client and was invited over to her house to obtain the signature if he still needed it today. He was overwhelmed.

~ ~ ~

"Allie, can you come to my office please?" Doc asked.

"Sure Doc, I'll be right there," I replied. As I ran down the stairs stepping over the garbage, I wondered *Now what did I do wrong?*

He began with a question, "You have never had a facet case have you?"

"No," I said. Facet means pregnant, I knew that at least.

"It's about time, I want you to handle this client. Open the chart and look at the physical. I started some of the initial clinical assessment for you."

"Thanks Doc, tell me about this client," I said taking the chart.

"Well, she is seven and a half months pregnant and just started prenatal care yesterday. Here is her Ob/Gyn report, the baby is already abnormal size. Job skills as a topless dancer; two other children living with her grandmother; recently widowed."

"Gee Doc, with a start like that we got nowhere to go but up, huh?"

"Good luck Allie, this is a tough one. Let me introduce you to her. " We went into the exam room, "Jaime, this is Allie, she is your counselor. I know you are not well, so you can talk to her tomorrow." Turning to me he said, "Allie, put a hold on her dose so you can do her intake properly, all right?"

This girl had the potential to be drop-dead gorgeous. She had normal heroin signs of wear and tear: a few abscess scars, a few knife wounds. She stood about five foot ten, had long blond hair, wide blue eyes, and not a sign of pregnancy under her sweats. At the end of her right arm was the most immaculate, precious, and angelic three-and-a-half year-old I have ever seen.

This blond ringlet-topped big blue-eyed girl who was pulling on my shirt said with a lisp, "I'm Cath, there's my baby si'ther," and she pointed to Jamie's stomach.

"Yeah, this is Cass," Jamie said, "She and this baby have the same father. He just died of an overdose. I have another daughter named Cory, she is five years old. Look, can I talk to you tomorrow? I am gonna be sick…" she barely managed to get out before covering her mouth.

"Okay, sure Jamie, tomorrow then," I wave her on.

~ ~ ~

It was 9:30AM and something was up. Javier was in the office with the doctor, Ethel, Moses, and Bonnie. Bonnie's face was red so I could tell she was mad. Everyone was told there would be an emergency counselor's meeting at lunch and it was mandatory that everyone be there at 10:00AM sharp, it should not be a long meeting.

I was still the new kid and was not one of the chosen few the boss would walk up to and say, "What do *you* think?" Any of the others might get this privilege, however, Javier was infamous for his inability to make a decision on his own. He was not even there half the time and when he was, it was chaos. The original Dr. Jekyll and Mr. Hyde, I never knew where I stood with him. I usually went to Jack for help since I had not quite made it into the trusted inner circle.

Everyone could get passionate about the clients, either for or against them. We had weekly meetings when it was decided by a vote if a client was eligible for take-homes. It was called a "Case Presentation." If it is done correctly, in my opinion, the client's name would not be mentioned. It would be "Number 6843 has a job evidenced by this paycheck stub or a letter from his employer, he has been on the program X number of days, and clean for such 'n such length of time." However, our case presentations were done by using names and most of the clients had been seen by each counselor, therefore, all the counselors knew their stories.

Sometimes, I saw more dysfunctional behavior with the staff at the clinic than in the clients. Whatever this meeting was about, it was hot. I was the last one in the room. Ethel, Angie, and Bonnie were all talking at the same time. Moses and Jack were talking together, the rest of the counselors were getting their food in front of them.

Bonnie spouted, "*She* should not be allowed on the program."

Angie and Joe both said at the same time, "No way will I take her for a client."

Ethel said, "Yeah, but she is MediCal and we cannot refuse her treatment."

Jack chimed in, "Oh yes we can!"

So I had to ask, "Who, what , when and where, what's up?"

"Linda!" they all chanted together.

Angie and Ethel voiced in harmony, "Allie can handle her!"

Jack stated, "That's not fair, she already has all the high-profile tough clients."

"Yes, but she can handle them," Doc added.

Boss Javier said, "Let's put it to a vote."

All talking at once, Bonnie interrupted, "You can't let her back."

"But she is MediCal," repeated Ethel and Angie in unison.

"So our life is worth an insurance claim?" Bonnie asked half-jokingly.

"We can't really refuse treatment," Javier flatly stated.

"So what is so bad about this client?" I finally spoke up, "before we vote and all."

Bonnie started with spit flying out of her mouth she was so mad, "Well, for one thing she is a paranoid schizophrenic with twelve different medications, constantly dirty, her husband suffers from PTSD (Post Traumatic Stress Disorder) and she threw her last counselor out the window! That is why she is seeking a new clinic."

"Sounds like her counselor must have pissed her off. I don't care, I'll take her," I said.

Jack chimed in again, "Allie, no really, that is not fair. She already hates me and I have never been tossed out a window before, it will be something to look forward to! How did we leave the situation with her?"

Javier stated, "I told her we would get back to her after lunch."

"Okay, is she still down there?" I asked. "Maybe I can get an idea before we commit, get a contract or something. Let me see how it goes. All in favor?"

The group agreed that if I thought I could handle her, she gets on; if the interview went bad, she was out of here. Bonnie and Moses abstained from voting.

So, down the stairs I went to face the most dramatic woman I had seen in a long time. She stood nicely dressed with carrot-red hair, purse on one arm and a hand resting on a cane. She looked like she was ready for war and either the cane or the purse would be the immediate weapon. I found out four months of pure hell later that the cane did have a knife at the bottom of it and she always kept a loaded gun in her purse! I do not know if those facts would have changed my approach to her had I known them, but I did not learn this until the week before her discharge, which at that point I encouraged.

It was not Linda that almost killed me, but Javier. The truth was he did not want her at the clinic, but was greedy. He also did not want to lose MediCal dollars or write up a report on why we refused her treatment. This *is* a business you know. This time with this client, my life took a twist into something that would take me a long time from which to recover.

"Those chicken-shit assholes sent you down here to get rid of me, didn't they?" she yelled with tears forming in the corners of her eyes. She continued in her best tough girl growling bulldog approach, "Well, I have rights goddamn it, you can't refuse me treatment, bitch."

I took a stance outside of the cane's reach, we were outside the clinic doors where there were always a bunch of people. I looked around to see who was there, they were all friendly. Most of the other clients were afraid of her too, you could tell. But I was far from alone, all the staff was upstairs watching through the window and the surrounding clients were frozen in time waiting to see what I would do.

I began, "If you will hold your tongue for a few, I am the only friend you have here right now. If I were you, I wouldn't piss-off the only chance you have to get on this program." I had an audience and I knew this could turn on me real fast.

Suddenly there were chants: "Hey, Allie's cool" "She's good man" "She'll work with you."

Linda's face changed, the tears were allowed to flow. I reached out my hand and said, "Hi, I am Allie. I might be your counselor."

"What do you mean *might* be my counselor?" she asked.

"It is up to you and me right now," I said calmly, "so do you want to go talk?"

As we stood there, I started to remember my internship where I conducted groups for rapists and murderers. It was at the California Youth Authority. The first day during group, all the inmates had to introduce themselves and state their crimes. They were all young men. Going around the circle they each reported: "I killed my mom," "I killed my stepfather," "I killed my stepmother," "I killed the real estate agent." They all seemed to make sense to me then, crimes of the heart, crimes of a child. I was dying to know why the one guy killed the real estate agent since that was how I was paying for school at the time! It was my curiosity that got me into trouble.

I now wanted to know why Linda threw her counselor out of the window! How does one get themselves into that sort of situation and how can I avoid it, right? Oh, by the way, the reason the kid killed the real estate agent was because his mom told him to and he did not want to piss-off his mother.

My reverie was interrupted when Linda said, "Sure, I'll talk."

We walked into the clinic, it was closed but the counselors remained upstairs. Moses was close by but not too close; security guard yes, crazy no. Linda went into the automatic story of her addiction which some at the clinic had memorized. To maximize our victimhood, we all know how to act when we need to and she was starting an award-winning performance.

I interrupted, "No, stop there. Why did you toss your last counselor out the window?"

She laughed.

I told her, "I don't think it is funny and neither does anyone else, that's why I am you're only hope to get on the program."

How she explained it was that it all came down to anger management, chemical imbalance, etc. The thing I respected most was when she said, "I need methadone more than I need to toss another counselor through a window and this is the closest clinic I can get to that I haven't been locked out of." That sentence was probably the most truthful thing I had heard all day.

I started in on the conditions: Keep a low profile (with her hair alone that was impossible); no loitering; do not talk to anyone but me; give me urine samples when I ask for them; and, just be invisible. I truly felt sorry for this lady, it was obvious she had been beautiful at one time. She was educated and despite what was going on presently, she had two children at home and lived with a crazy man. Crazy husbands lead to crazy women, this I know to be true.

I tried to make Linda my friend, I sure as hell did not want her as my enemy. She was very smart, she had worked in the medical field at one time. I cannot remember exactly which field but she had the terminology down. I imagine she could manipulate any doctor into just about anything, so could most of the clients, but she was really good at it.

I learned that afternoon that Linda's husband had been a Vietnam veteran. She told me they were going through some tests because her husband had been exposed to Agent Orange. They were also working with the children for chromosome damage. They went to the VA hospital twice a week, that is where her husband got his methadone.

Things were going smooth with Linda until the need for her first prescription approval. I tried to explain how the program worked and that if she wanted to fight the system's politics, to do it correctly. She continued to compare our program with the rules for the VA hospital, I tried to explain it was not the same.

Then she wanted take-homes.

"No can do," I said. Well, that pissed her off. I told her we needed to argue her point the right way, there were ways to appeal.

When I got called in to Javier's office to discuss Linda's phone call to the State of California and another call from our auditor with MediCal who was asking questions about why our client was contacting his office, I just laughed. Javier did not think this was funny.

I told him, "I sure as heck did not tell her to call anyone. I simply stated to her that there was a correct way to challenge the system and an incorrect way; for example, tossing a counselor out the window."

I suggested to him that we were making progress in her rehabilitation. I think he really had it in for this woman, or me. I did not know which of us he was more upset with, or why.

~ ~ ~

"Hi, this is Jaime. You have a hold on my dose."

I said, "Oh, good afternoon Jamie, can you come upstairs for a little while?"

She stated that she really was not feeling well, that she did not think her dose was holding and already wanted an increase. I asked again if she could make it upstairs.

She said she had Cass with her.

I said, "Great."

Jamie began telling me that both her children were born on methadone and she knew what she was doing. "Look at her, she looks normal doesn't she?" she asked, pointing to her daughter.

She certainly did seem okay. She was well mannered, assertive, and attempting to demonstrate her abilities of charm and intelligence with the letters she was drawing for me.

"I know what I am doing," she continued. "I mean my life is a mess but my kids are okay."

I asked if she could stay; she asked to do it tomorrow. I explained that the dose increase must come from her Ob/Gyn. She was not happy about that but would go today to see him anyway.

The next day with her dose hold in place, Jamie again begged out of the session and for more methadone. Everyone was reluctant to adjust methadone in the third trimester, for good reason. The continued sickness after one week told me she was still using. I had just obtained her intake urine test results and there was not much she and her baby were not taking. The results showed cocaine, heroin, codeine, and amphetamine; on top of this, she smoked one and a half packs of cigarettes a day, and drank lots of coffee. But she is not a drinker, she reported.

After nine days of avoidance, Jamie finally sat down with me. I had been in her face every day since she got here, at least she appeared to be gaining weight.

"Oh, Allie, I got a prescription for some T-3s," she said.

I said, "For what?"

"T-3s, you know, Tylenol with codeine #3," she continued that she had to get her tooth pulled yesterday.

"Does your dentist know you are pregnant?" I asked.

"Hell no, he never would have taken me!"

I started to remember the way things were way-back-when and of calling my doctor to ask if I could take an *aspirin* when I was pregnant! I confronted her with her urine test results. She had no explanation other than that is why she was here.

"I got real worried because I did a lot of speed in the beginning of this pregnancy," Jamie stated. "I wasn't sure if I was going to keep the baby or not. But then I got to thinking about my husband dying and little Cass and all. It would be her full-blooded sister and all."

Jamie continued to relate the story of when her husband had just gotten out of jail. He had been clean for a while but like any addict, all he could think about was a fix. She had been working when he got out, she met with him on a break just long enough to get pregnant, her words. When she returned home, he was dead with a needle still in his arm. She said that she freaked-out for a while. But then she met a very nice widower at the cemetery while visiting her husband's grave who had lots of money and wanted to help her.

The next day she came to the clinic she was driving a brand new forty-thousand dollar automobile. I got a buzz on the intercom from Jack stating that I needed to go check out the new ride my client had, and he wanted details. Since there was now a permanent hold on her dose, getting details would not be a problem. I had many requirements to complete before Jamie's baby was born and we knew most likely the baby would come early, so there was no time to spare. Besides, I had to keep as close an eye on her as I could for the baby's sake.

I said, "Nice new car."

"Yeah, my little honey-bunny got it for me. He wanted me to come over last night and my grandma would not let me use her car. So when I got up this morning, it was in the driveway," she explained with a big smile.

[Note: I relayed to Jack this new information; he wanted to know if she would take checks.]

Jamie continued her story saying she was fourteen when she first used heroin. She said she still wondered if the teacher who found her in the junior high bathroom shooting-up had ever recovered. She was ten years old when her parents separated, her father moved to the valley and her mother moved to Hawaii. She hung out at the beach and was in the process of becoming a champion level surfer.

However, Jamie's mother had a real agenda with surfers, telling her that they were all heroin addicts. She also told Jamie if she continued to associate with them, she would become one. Jamie admitted that surfing was just something you cannot give up, especially when you lived at the beach.

Her mother finally gave up the battle and told her, "One more time with that crowd and you will go live with your grandmother."

Jaime looked at me straight in the eyes and said, "I swear to you none of the people I hung out with did drugs. We were all health nuts trying to be the next sponsored surfer and I was a good one too. My life would be so different if mom hadn't forced me to move in with my grandma. I don't think my mom knew there was so much drug use in this area. It only took me one week after moving out here to find it. I went straight for the heroin, the first drug I ever used, just to spite my mom. I was sent to rehab after the teacher found me but I have used on and off ever since. I know how to use my looks and get what I want."

Jamie continued on her roller coaster life, if she did not find trouble, it found her. Due to the fact that she was pregnant, we were required to test her weekly. I do not think there was one clean test. Somehow when the baby was born at eight and a half months, she was clean and so was the baby, they went home together. The baby appeared to be healthy, it sure was big.

Jaime had her honey-bunny wrapped around her little finger. When I saw her after the birth of her baby there was not a trace that she had just delivered a nearly nine-pound infant. New clothes, new dreams. Honey-bunny was going to set her up in an apartment so she could live with her children. She was spending most of her time attempting to be a mother, and of course, shopping for furniture.

A few details Jaime neglected to tell me was that she was on parole and she had no driver's license. The newborn was about two months old when Jamie came running up the stairs into my office and asked if I had a minute. I had not seen her up close in two weeks. She had complied with all the necessary requirements in the program but she looked horrible. She was obviously on a drug-run and it looked like crack.

My first response when she walked in the room was, "You look like hell!"

She said she had taken up the pipe to lose baby fat.

I asked, "What baby fat?"

She said, "I have blown it, I am in big trouble."

Jamie had discovered that honey-bunny had a daughter her age and she was not happy with their relationship. She continued, "I got pulled over for speeding and my charm was not working. The officer asked for my license. I told him I had left my wallet at home."

Jamie gave the officer the name and address of honey-bunny's daughter. She told me if she had admitted that she had no license it would be a misdemeanor but the lie she told could be a felony, she did not know what to do. Her biggest fear was that she had just blown her meal ticket with honey-bunny.

Shortly after that, Jaime was on her way back to prison. The baby was allowed to stay with her sisters which was a good thing based on what I had observed. It was about six months later that Jaime was back at the clinic strung-out on heroin.

"When did you get out?" I asked her.

"Yesterday," she replied.

I asked, "How?"

"It's who you know. I couldn't do all this time without drugs and they're easy to get inside," she said flippantly.

I remember the first time I discovered flaws in our rehabilitation system. I was doing my internship at the California Youth Authority, the prisoners had the right to refuse drug testing. It was a cost, but one I guess they were willing to pay. Many of the clients had expressed how easy it was to get drugs in prison, just about anything you wanted. "Where there is a will, there is a way" they would say. Just one more reminder of what a joke the "war on drugs" campaign really was.

Jaime indicated she had taken classes while doing her time and she had dreams of working again. It was not long before she drove-up in her new car again, I guess honey-bunny was not mad anymore. Then in another couple of weeks she looked like she was using methamphetamine again, the cycle of the working girl.

One day, I had a hold on Jamie for a counseling session. She said she could not wait because her probation officer was in his car waiting for her and that he could put her back into prison in any time if she did not do what he said.

I looked at her and asked, "What does he want?"

She so casually replied, "A blowjob will keep him happy."

I said in disbelief, "Get out of here!"

"Really, he is out in the car waiting."

I walked out with her and a male was sitting in a plain car. She jumped in with him and did some animated talking while pointing at me, they took off. I just stood there.

Jack walked up and asked me, "What's up?"

I told him that Jaime could not stay for her counseling session because she had to give her parole officer a blowjob.

He said, "It's probably true, and if not, it's one hell of a good excuse to get out of a session!"

9 | Conflicts Within the System

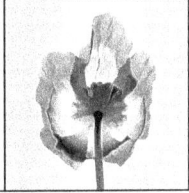

Changes were coming in the Social Security programs. Most of the clinic's clients had been classified permanently disabled due to their addiction. They had obtained Social Security benefits that were soon to be terminated, unless they could prove they were indeed disabled and receiving regular medical attention. Simply being on methadone would no longer qualify them.

Many of the clients did have serious medical and psychological needs but they had their methadone, and everything else was fine when you inquired. Most of the medical and/or psychological issues that were disabling them were put off since a monthly check arrived and the methadone bill was paid. Getting to the doctor was always going to be tomorrow or next week, there was always a good reason the appointment had to be canceled. This was why I frequently took my clients across the street to Dr. Chan. She was very helpful and we worked well together.

Javier began the discussion, "You are all aware of the pending changes in Social Security and the potential consequences of those stated changes. So, if you want to keep your jobs, I suggest that you assist your clients with the required forms. The information I have received from our corporate office states that the clients should be receiving them in the mail this week and they should be returned with supporting documentation by the end of next month. I expect each one of you will be able to help your clients in ascertaining the retention of their benefits."

Bonnie spoke up and asked, "Just exactly what does that mean?"

Javier retorted, "I don't expect to lose one MediCal client over this. Is that clear enough for you?"

The conversations started buzzing. Venting began regarding the freeloaders sucking-up our tax dollars and our retirement futures or even our jobs, all this enveloped the room. Can you imagine the conflict?

Jack spoke above the noise, "Hell, it's no different than referring them to the attorneys we did four years ago to get the damn benefits to begin with. You remember that don't you Bonnie?"

"I don't know," she stated, "this sounds like fraud."

"What do you mean fraud?" shouted Javier.

"Oh never mind," she said.

Well, the forms started to arrive and the clients panicked. We told them what to expect and that we would help, but all they could focus on was "How will I live without my methadone?" I guess their rent did not worry them.

The next problem was that psychological evaluations were required and none of us were qualified to perform them. During the next meeting, Javier inquired if any of us had a psychiatrist in our pocket or knew of one that would effectively do the job. We found one who wanted three hundred dollars per client upfront, or at least after interviewing them all. The corporate office gave the approval and we embarked on the task of trying to rope-in the clients to keep their money coming in.

I thought it would be easy for the clients, all they had to do was show up at a certain time, answer a few questions and *poof* they get free money and free methadone. Some of the clients just needed to fill out the forms and put them in the mail. Many claimed to have never received them, but that was okay, we could give them a set when they arrived. Clients made several phone calls attempting to obtain their medical documentation, and lots of appointments were made.

Mind you, in the past we were not allowed to do this or that for a client, but now we were to do *everything* for them from arranging taxis to filling out forms; from taking the client to medical appointments to standing in line at the Social Security Office. Oh, how policies change when money is involved!

The shrink was at the clinic for three days and saw most of our clients. One group session I will never forget because I have never laughed so hard. It was four men who usually rode together that were going to have their evaluations together— don't even ask. We directed them to wait in our lunch-room. Their average age was forty-five but they were like thirteen-year-old boys in detention.

This group of troublemakers had the forms and were adlibbing the answers. I wish I had a video recorder, there was so much spontaneous, dark humor. They even tried to sneak smoking cigarettes, getting into the refrigerator, and sneak out entirely! One of them asked me if masturbation during the interview would score points. They pretended to mumble to imaginary pets and friends, it was just controlled insanity. It was hilarious to me at the time!

The funniest of this bunch was actually a guy who was seriously disabled. At one time, he was the most dangerous of criminals. He would never be serious with me when I asked him about his crimes. He was not my client but I gave him a ride to the dentist anyway. Call it animal instinct but I knew he would never hurt me, protect me was more like it. I only threw this face around a few times, but I had some pretty strong connections to various gangs in the area. I was their friend. It seems funny now, but *this* ex-PTA President had some real bad homeboys and homegirls she could call on if needed.

Jack used his similar connections once. His stepdaughter had been living with a guy he never liked and she called home one day telling him that the boyfriend had beaten her up. She wanted to come home but the guy would not let her take her belongings and even hid her car keys. Jack had been at the clinic for a few years when this occurred so he called one of his clients, "You said if I ever needed anything, well…"

That same day five of the meanest ugliest bad boys met Jack at his stepdaughter's apartment. They knocked on the door and when the boyfriend opened it the biggest guy was in his face saying, "We are here to move Donna, do you want to help or get hurt?" She was moved out without a problem.

~ ~ ~

Sometimes getting on "the system" or being on "the system" did more damage than good. One client I really liked was Mary. She was my age and had grown up in the same area as I did. She had some physical problems but the worst addiction was her choice in men. She was very smart. Most of our sessions were intelligent conversations, that is, when she was not crying the blues about the last domestic scene. We talked about how she could get out of her abusive rut. She had more of a problem with alcohol than heroin; but both of these drugs, did not compare to the *man drug* to which she was addicted.

I shared with her in celebration of her stability and dose tapering and I almost had her off the program. I also shared with her the worst of her bottoming-out, at least for which I was aware. I was introduced to her mother, sister, and niece; I even had her s/o on my caseload. He was a nice guy, they were just a bad couple. We often reminded ourselves at the clinic: One can only rise to the lowest level of a relationship while on drugs or alcohol.

Mary trusted me so much that she brought her family to me for help. I gave it my best, but too much had to change in her family. I had three generations of liquor-lovers in my office at one time; Mary's niece at only fourteen years old with a drinking problem, and her mother and sister. I earned Mary's respect about two months after she started coming to the clinic. I always told my clients that I would be there for them if they needed me. I had no idea I would be tested so soon with Mary.

Mary apparently had a bad Friday night with the significant other. She had come to the clinic early that morning and pleaded with the counselor of the weekend to call me at home. The counselor refused stating that whatever it was it could wait until Monday. Mary also pleaded for my phone number and was bluntly refused. Mary being Mary, she magically produced my business card and called everyone in the phone book with my last name! As it turned out, I kept my first husband's name due to the fact that my two daughters were so young at the time of our divorce.

Mary eventually found my ex-husband's phone number and called him at home. It was 9:30AM Saturday morning. I was at home just finishing the breakfast dishes when I got the call, "Allie, I just got a very distressing phone call," my ex-husband announced.

"Really?" I replied. Immediately I thought something was up with the girls.

"Apparently, one of your clients is in desperate need of speaking with you. She explained that she went through the phonebook calling everyone with our last name asking if they knew you and how to get in touch with you. I told her that I knew you and that I would call you. She said that if you could not call she would understand, but she sounds desperate. Here is her phone number."

Remember, this was the same man who would not shake my hand after he found out where I was working! I thanked him on her behalf and pardoned the interruption of his morning. For the first time since I had known him, he sounded respectful of my abilities and truly concerned.

I dialed the number he gave me and Mary picked-up the phone crying. She knew right away it was me when I said, "Is this you Mary?"

She recalled the story of how she found me, the story of her saga, her apologies and her understanding if I refused to help her—like I could refuse. She and the s/o had gotten into what I was about to learn was a routine battle. She wanted to leave him and go into a shelter, she was sure this is what she wanted. I think if I could have found a shelter or home for her, the story would have had a different ending. I called every shelter from San Bernardino to Orange and Los Angeles Counties, not one would consider taking someone on methadone. [Note: One year later, I tried to help a social worker find a residence for one of my senior citizens from the clinic, we could not find an assisted living facility to take a methadone client then either.]

I called Mary back and explained I could not find anywhere that would take her due to being on methadone. She could, however, start the process of detox-ification and go into the hospital for a thirty-day stay and get clean. This was not the solution to her homeless situation that night, besides, she had gone the hospit-al route before and would not consider going back. Mary said, "You are witnessing the success of that hospital program choice!"

We both laughed and I said, "At least you still have your sense of humor."

"So do you," she laughed.

She stayed at her mother's house Saturday night and by Monday she and the s/o were back together. Mary did real well for a long while, then came the slide. She was not at her best when the psychological evaluation was needed and at the end of her session the psychologist asked if I were her counselor.

"Yes, it's a shame isn't it?" I said.

"You do know Mary is more intelligent than you or I or your Director here, don't you? Let me show you," he said as he retrieved some papers from his desk.

Javier being the idiot that he could be said, "Great, Doc, I wanted to see what you do to get three hundred dollars per client!"

The doctor asked Javier three questions and showed him three pictures. After receiving Javier's answers, he said, "Mary outscored you by 200 points." I got the feeling he did not like Javier.

For several weeks after the evaluations were completed, we tried to reach the psychologist by phone. We needed the reports but he would not return our phone calls. Then one day Todd (White Todd) called his answering service stating he was suicidal to try to get a response. The doctor returned that phone call. Obviously, he was not pleased with Todd's methodology.

As it turned out, he had not sent the reports because Javier had not sent his check yet. However, we did not lose too many people due to the system changes and the ones we lost still came to the clinic, they just paid out-of-pocket.

~ ~ ~

When Linda's car pulled up, Moses, the security guard called me. I had to be with her just about the entire time she was on the property, and the truth was she was not doing a damn thing different from anyone else. In my opinion, she was being singled out. Javier was acting erratic, there was no consistency in his attitude or behavior. Several of us were beginning to wonder if he were using drugs! We found out the answer to Javier's erratic behavior about two years later.

In the meantime, Linda had requested a meeting with him several days ago but he simply ignored her. Several times I was told I better keep my client under control. Then one day, when her polite requests were ignored and her telephone calls went unanswered, she walked back into the doctor's office and requested to speak with him. Bad timing, he was not in his best of moods and freaked-out calling me on the loudspeaker to come to his office because my client was there.

I had no idea anything was going on. I grabbed her chart and came down just as though there was a medical problem. I got downstairs and the doctor yelled at me for not controlling my client. He told me he already had called Javier; and when he arrived, yelled at him too.

At this point, I took Linda aside and suggested today was not a good day to pursue her agenda. I suggested that she get in her car and go home. She did get in her car and I went up the stairs to my office. However, when I was out of sight, Linda had gotten out of her car and marched up the opposite staircase to Javier's office. Our offices were at opposite ends of the building. I had just sat down when I heard both Javier and Linda's voices shouting out my name. I jumped-up and ran down the hall. The three of us jammed in the doorway, Linda had her purse and cane in hand. Like any predator in survival mode, she could smell his fear and was going for the kill.

Linda was criticizing the amount of time Javier was not at the clinic (okay, so he was never there, but we liked it that way!). Then she commented about his alleged affair with the dosing nurse and congratulated him on how her baby looked so much like him.

Linda added, "And by the way, what does the nurse's husband think about the resemblance?"

"Allie, your client and her mouth is going to force me to call the police if you cannot control her," Javier shouted. He fell into her trap, he lost control.

I found out all she wanted was clarification on why she could not get take-homes. The Director of the clinic at the VA hospital had suggested to Linda some things to discuss with the Director at her clinic. So she was actually trying to play by the rules. I took her by the shoulders, looked her in the eyes and said, "Would you please come down to my office, *now*."

She said, "I am trying to fight for my rights the right way."

"I know, but this is not a good time. Please for me, can we go to my office?" I asked while nudging her out the doorway. We left and that was when I learned of the loaded gun in her purse and the knife in her cane. She did not show them to me but I did not need to see them to believe her.

I spent a good half an hour with her, she had a legitimate request and complaint. We talked about choices and consequences and that she was really in a bad situation and this was not helping her. She agreed to leave and to start look-ing for an alternative clinic.

After that day, I had all the clinic's staff support concerning Linda's situation, with the exception of Javier. The other counselors came in and told me that if I wanted to file charges of emotional distress due to job stress, they would back me up.

Actually, the stress of these few months when Linda was on my caseload, in addition to all the others, was taking its toll on me physically. Soon after Linda's tyrant, she disappeared. We started a dose taper order just in case of her return. I felt her dose was low enough that she could utilize her endless prescriptions of medication to prevent withdrawal symptoms. It just makes you wonder how many Lindas there are trying to resolve conflicts within "the system."

10 Killing Time

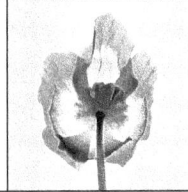

I was told that Yolanda was a real problem client. Evidently, she always came to dose right before closing for lunch; she never cooperated during sessions; she frequently threw temper tantrums; her urine testing was a nightmare and she needed to be watched very closely. The first time I met Yolanda, it went well.

"You have seven children?" I asked.

"Yes," she said.

"I would use drugs too if I had seven kids!" I kidded back. "How do you do it?"

I learned that her mother actually had legal custody of all seven children and she lived with her and the kids. However, now her mom could not take care of the children and Yolanda did not want them to end up like she and her sister. Yolanda related that Social Services did not know of the arrangement with her mother and could not find out. This was a typical situation with Child Protective Services. As my friend Moses would say, "It makes you wonder just what is really going on."

Where was the logic in keeping the family together other than less paperwork? If the mom had raised two heroin addicted females who in turn produced children, what made this family think things would be different for the grandchildren? Sure it was better than Foster Care, sometimes, or maybe not. As with Jane's children, *comadre* is a word that means godmother, it does not mean blood relative. Jane's kids were taken away and look what happened to her! Regardless of how abusive Jane may or may not have been, I just know she did not kill her son.

Three out of four weeks, Yolanda was a relatively pleasant person. She had to report her agenda with the staff at the clinic. The nurses hated her. She would spout allegations of sexual misconduct with Director Javier and Black Todd. She also suggested that the clinic doctor was a quack. Yolanda was a miserable person with a miserable life. She worked on and off but the truth was with seven children with seven school schedules, how could she work and keep up with them all? Most of the women at the clinic with children have been hounded-to-death by someone to obtain employment, I guess the concept was to get them off Welfare. In most cases, I did not agree.

I had been able to control Yolanda most of the time but either her tantrums got worse or my patience wore thin. It was during the time just before Linda left that Yolanda was pushing everyone's buttons, including mine. I discussed it at the counselor's meeting, and much to my surprise, they agreed that if I could not handle her nobody else could. So, if I wanted her thrown off the program, I had not only support but encouragement!

I called Yolanda upstairs to discuss her behavior and how it had to change. I attempted to give her an out and tried to reestablish communication by asking if there was a problem, or if she wanted another counselor? It did not go well, she stormed out of my office without a word. The next day, I put a hold on her dose. She would be given a contract about her possible termination. She had a fit of rage with the dispensing nurse and as the doctor walked by, she threw a few foul words in his direction. She was all fired-up when I appeared.

"You fucking bitch, get that goddamn hold off my dose. I saw you yesterday," she yelled.

I looked at the dispensing nurse then at Yolanda and said, "You can come back for your dose with a different attitude at 12:25PM." It was 9:50AM.

She went-off again and I suggested she leave now, before any other action took place. Moses had his hand on the phone ready to call the police.

With her final "fuck you," I told her that her transfer papers would be waiting when she called. She got in her car and never came back.

So one easygoing counselor, me, just kicked a client off the program! I waited for retribution, you know it is coming you just never know when. As it turned out, nobody questioned my decision and none of the clients ever mentioned it either. My call was justified, Yolanda had blown it.

~ ~ ~

Steve was a hard case. He had been on the program for almost a year when he was assigned to me but had a history at the clinic that went back several years. Steve's father, at one time, was on the program. Jack had his dad on his caseload and he had nothing but contempt for Steve. I had not discovered this until the day I mentioned to Jack that I was stuck with a client and did not know which way to go with him.

Steve rarely had more than an "I 'm just fine, thank you" to say to me. He was on 60 milligrams and obviously the eightball or speedball was his drug of choice, he had never had a clean test. I tried to get a conversation going with him but it was impossible.

Well, the clinic had the computer setup so that on a client's birthday, the Happy Birthday song would chime on cue. Steve was producing a urine sample for me as I had just cleared his name for dosing when he came walking out of the restroom with his bottle. As I wished him a Happy Birthday along with the computer, I inquired what were his celebration plans.

"I am a dope fiend, what the hell do you think my plans are?" he barked.

"Watch the attitude or I'll bake you a cake for next year," I said and got him to smile a bit. It was a first!

I later shared this information with Jack and his response was really nasty. "Why waste time on that asshole, he is scum of the earth. He pimps the mother of his children, in fact, he set her up to give his dad a blowjob when he was in the hospital last time. He treats his mother like dirt and does nothing but drive whores and shoplifters around to commit crimes. Don't waste your time."

Once when I got Steve in my office for a session, he was very honest with me. He stated that he was just "killing time" until he died. He drank a six-pack of beer a day and used as much as he could afford. He told me a dose increase would just make him use more when he went on fee detox.

"Just don't waste my time, or yours," he said.

"You are the second person to say that to me about you, but then why are you here?" I asked him.

"I can't afford the habit," he replied.

I thanked him for his honesty. Eventually, there were changes. He actually started to spend some time with his son. During this time, he claimed life was grand until he found out the boy's mother was using heroin and prostituting during the day. This was when Steve turned to *the life*. I think I got one or two clean tests out of him, and heck, I thought a smile was progress. Then he started a relationship with a woman client at the clinic and seemed to be doing okay.

On his next birthday, to prove he had plans, Steve brought his son in to meet me so I would not bake him a "damn cake." I did give him a card though. Soon after his birthday, the woman client he had been living with called to tell me that Steve was in the hospital. He was having uncontrolled diabetic problems and his liver was failing. She was not sure if he was going to make it. I called him at the hospital and reminded him to be nice, that was the last I spoke or heard from

Steve.

~ ~ ~

The only thing I was told about Joanne was that she would not get a job. Joanne was my age but looked ten years older. During our first session she stated, "I am not going to get a job until my youngest gets out of school."

"Fine with me," I said. "How about getting off methadone then?"

I think she would have rather gotten a job. She had been on the program for forever and was clean. No one had tried to get her take-homes. She was taking care of her children and grandchildren. Joanne had no interest other than keeping her kids off the streets which she said was a full-time job, I agreed. Most of the clients lived in the jungle, most of the people around them were animals. Money does not breed evil, it is the lack of money that breeds evil. I support stay-at-home moms as long as they were mothering.

I set Joanne up for take-homes and she promised to see a doctor regarding her female health problems, I suggested to her the possibly of menopause. She stated that her mother had told her the same thing and she had not gone to a doctor in years. She did not want to get the exam with our doctor. I did not blame her and remarked, "I would not have my manicurist do my bikini waxing either!" She agreed to see Dr. Chan.

It was one hell of a battle with the initial take-home for Joanne but with a little help from Jack who I had to convince, she got them. Her personality lifted slightly after this. No longer the depressed victim who was wrong for what she thought was right, she actually had someone in her corner. I could not get Joanne to budge on tapering her dose initially, then eventually talked her into a blind dose. A *blind dose* is when a client promises to not ask the milligrams per dose and the nurses do not reveal the dose strength. This takes mega-trust, as well as, the client's need to address their psychological addictions.

I had to *prove* psychological addiction to Joanne, there were just some things I could not teach her. The first time she agreed to a dose taper, I got a gut feeling what I should do. I believe in intuition and have always lived by it. I told her I would process her dose, but I did not actually change the milligram strength.

One week after our discussion of the blind dose taper, Jane came to me and said, "I can't take it! I am in withdrawal. My bones hurt, I have diarrhea, I have the sweats all the time, and I feel the need to use for the first time in years."

"That is menopause," I said flatly.

"It is not, it is withdrawal," she tried to convince me.

"It can't be, because I did not touch your dose level," I revealed. "Did you go see the doctor like you promised?"

She said, "No."

"Do you believe in women's intuition?"

"Yes," she replied.

"I had a *feeling* you would react this way," I told her.

I printed out her dosing sheets for the last thirty days to prove there had been no dose changes. We had a good laugh together. She went to the doctor for her exam and I started a very slow taper about a month later. Joanne was a great client. She came to see me on her own, followed all the rules, was low profile, had no issues with Social Services or Parole—no problems period. Then I gave her space. She was already doing the one thing I wanted her to do, get off the program.

Sadly, the morning came when I arrived at the clinic and Joanne was sitting in the back of a police car, handcuffed. The officers were polite enough to allow me to speak with her, she was a wreck. She was able to talk to me because the clinic had not yet opened. In between her tears, she told me the story.

It seemed her son had been in the company of two boys who were accused of robbing an ice-cream vendor in the park. She had been there when she saw the police roughing up the boys. She screamed out, "If you hurt my son, I will kill you." Something any mother would say, don't you think? Well, the police arrested her for being a terrorist threat! But as I mentioned earlier, it was a jungle out there.

Joanne spent twelve days in jail and was given three years parole. If she did anything, as she put it, "farted sideways," she would do life. This was her third strike. Was she bitter? Who wouldn't be? I gave her space and tried to help her, but at this point she did not care.

Her son was innocent, the other boys confessed. Joanne said, "He got to do time for being in the wrong place at the wrong time." He received six months in a boy's detention camp. Everything Joanne had tried to avoid had happened. Neither he nor Joanne was ever the same. She tried to get him started again in school but he just asked, "Why?" Joanne could not give him an answer.

~ ~ ~

Elena was something else, she was bright and so full of optimism. She dressed in the most colorful clothing, all reds, yellows, and bright blues. Not my style but you always knew when Elena arrived! She was private pay and that meant on and off the program, and most likely had gone through a few counselors. She was transferred to me due to a conflict with her last counselor. I never did get the details, it could have been a momentary thing. She was a born-again Christian and had spent some time in a local Christian Home. She had been clean and sober for a few months.

Elena stated she had done some spiritual counseling and her pastor was encouraging her to create a program for women on methadone, she was trying to put it together. We talked about what being a counselor entailed and this communication worked as a backdoor approach to her treatment which, of course, she did not really need. She knew everything and had her life under control.

One of the things Elena wanted for herself and asked me to consider was to start a women's group at our clinic. I was shocked myself that we did not have one, as well as, several other group topics like 12 Step meetings. I asked the other counselors about it and was told no one would go to groups. Then I started questioning the clients. If I threw the party, would they come? The response was overwhelming. Javier did not care and the doctor was behind me one hundred percent.

Only two women attended the first meeting, but each week there were more eager participants showing up. I found I needed to get one successful group before I started a second or third. Soon, I was up to eight women and it was working! We were talking about real issues, real problems, and calling each other on their stories. The one stipulation I made was that they were not to focus on their addiction, but instead about being a woman and mother.

I will never forget one meeting when we were talking about seeing or not seeing their children while incarcerated, when Javier opened the door and said, "I need some spoons. Allie, do you know where the spoons are? Hey, someone get the spoons, you guys got any spoons on you?"

We all froze, considering spoons were a part of most drug paraphernalia! He found the box of spoons and laughing solo, he left the room.

I took a very long deep breath and said, "Now, where were we?" I tried to ignore how red my face looked.

Marty said, "That was rude."

Several others confirmed her statement by starring directly at me.

"Well!" I said as I tried to hold a snicker because they knew the corner I was now occupying. If I said anything of substance or of sarcastic quality, it would be the buzz of the clinic in an hour. So I replied, "Mama said if you can't say anything nice, don't say anything at all! I think you were talking Eleanor, please go on."

They snickered and let it go. It was awful and I do not think Javier had a clue for a long while what he had actually done. We were forced to discontinue the group shortly after Linda arrived. Javier thought we were using the time to talk about him to create a conspiracy or something. But I could not do it anymore anyway, it was just too much tension.

Elena had come from out-of-state about three years ago. She did not have a car but she did have a motorhome! She always drove it to the clinic and if the traffic issues in our parking lot were not bad enough, you can imagine what a motorhome did. The other scary thing about the motorhome was she kept three or four dogs in it. Because I allowed her to take my parking place, there were times this issue upset me more than the other counselors. Sometimes she would spend the night right there in the lot! How convenient, right? It took about three days of the motorhome not moving before I decided it could not be parked there any longer.

Then Elena had a falling out with the pastor over drinking and was asked to leave the home for a while. Even with all this turmoil, she mustarded-up the energy to follow through with her dream and her passion, the goal was evident. She had actually gone to a school and gathered information to get formal counseling training. The setback of being kicked-out of the church home was enough to push her into giving up.

When someone is weakened, their self-esteem becomes fragile. So at this point, Elena gave up the idea of becoming a counselor and this hit her hard. She was also losing another brother to AIDS and she asked for a temporary dosing request out-of-state to go visit him. Not a problem, we set it up and she had enough take-homes to get her where she was going. She would be able to dose for a while at a clinic out-of-state which was familiar to her. And, I got my parking space back.

Elena came back to the program after an extended visit of almost a month accompanied by the love of her life, in fact, they were married. He was an alcoholic and addict, with HIV complications. Full of marital bliss and renewed optimism, she wanted to pick up where she left off but she had more problems now, including the *man drug*. She was working at reestablishing herself with the pastor and trying to push her husband into her agenda without much success.

Soon Elena exhibited signs of not doing well, domestic violence was now incorporated into the drinking and drug abuse, a common threesome. The logic of happiness just did not add up to domestic bliss while they were living with the dogs in the motor home which was frequently parked in our lot, or to be exact, my parking space.

Sometimes, it was so easy to see from the outside looking in. As with most women, instead of focusing on herself or taking care of herself, Elena now focused all her attention on him—what he does, what he does not do, what he can do, what he will not do, etc. Then there were the battles and the painful disappointments which, of course, always required medicating.

Elena could not hear, could not see, and could not *be* because of her inability to control her life. Many lives out of control that could be disguised with a drink, a fix, or a pill often ended here. For most dependent women, the situation seemed the same. It was so amazing to watch these women. Even with hearing their own stories being repeated between them and reflecting on their mothers, sisters, and girlfriend's lives, they did not get it. They could even acknowledge these men were bad for them, yet they stayed with them anyway. I had never seen such unconditional love. When their men go to jail or prison, these women cleanup their lives. They get jobs, their children go to school and church, and just when they are reaching true stability, the husband or s/o gets released and the dominance starts all over again.

We have all had fantasies of being loved and having someone to love. I think that is why there are so many babies within this population. Too much was going against these women, like their history which could not be forgotten and the endless poverty. They lived in a society that stated it had opportunities for all, but continued to label and keep down those who were already down. It just took too much strength to succeed, it was just too hard.

"Why change?" they would declare. "It's the way it's been, it's all we know."

Like all the couples in the program, the cycle of two dependent hurting people continued to be love-fight-fix, love-fight-fix… So the bliss of immediate gratification through medication also cycled while they were just "killing time."

| 11 | Rays of Hope | 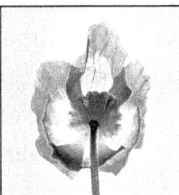 |

Annie was one of those women who managed to do some things right, she had finished high school for one thing and did not get pregnant before she graduated. These two accomplishments were significant and rare in this population. She did end up marrying the boy next door who was the bad boy, she worked and he played.

Annie was pregnant with her second child and working two jobs when a light came on and she realized her man should be doing something more than what he was doing, which was nothing except using heroin. She had no idea he was using at this time, she just thought he was lazy. He always had a reason for losing his job or not looking for work, but she was tired and cranky and his stories were just not working anymore. She left him and moved back into her parent's home for the sake of her children, her sanity, and to get some relief.

Annie had never been around heroin use and did not know the evident signs. She had been pretty naïve about drinking and drugs since she had come from a sober Christian family. When she discovered he was using and in an effort to understand it, as in many of the stories I heard, one night she asked him, "Can I try it to see what the big deal is?"

No one ever takes drugs thinking they will become addicted and Annie claims she was not for a long time but then it became her pain management. All good times must end and it did when her husband was arrested. Annie explained to her parents and they were supportive of her as long as he would no longer be in the picture and that she would get treatment.

Many factors go into the possibility of success for someone to reclaim their life after heroin. Annie possessed many of these factors. She started using the drug at an older age; it was not in her family; she had no legal history; she had a high school diploma; and, she had a successful employment history. Also, Welfare was not an accepted way of survival in her family and she had tremendous emotional support. So when she transferred to the clinic she declared, "I want off methadone as soon as possible. I have a life to live." I thought *Whoopee!*

Annie was on a low dose and had already been on the program for a year when I met her. She was working part-time and still living at home with her parents. We talked repeatedly about what she was going to do when or if her husband was released and, of course, she said he was not even a factor to consider. During the course of time on the program, even getting past the death of her father, she remained clean and continued with the dose tapering. Annie was my first client to detox off the program which was almost unheard of.

I heard about Annie once in a while because she had a friend at the clinic, someone who understood why they could not be friends anymore. Then about six months after she had been off the program, I saw her car in the parking lot. It was early and she was in the passenger seat. She was not real happy to see me when I walked up to the car and said, "Long time no see."

Shamefully, Annie looked up and said, "Allie, this is my husband. I need to get him on the program."

I intuitively felt this when I first approached their car. I tried to put on my best team-spirited smile. I directed my gaze to him and said, "Sure, I don't think there will be a problem. Why don't you go get in line? First come first served, you know."

This would give me a chance to tell Annie what I was really thinking which was *What the hell did you do? Are you out of your frigg'n mind?*

As it turned out, I did not get a chance to say a word to her. After the car door closed and he was three steps away she stated, "I know what you are going to say. So I put down the ground rules; he must be on the program, clean, and have a job by next Monday. I am clean and not using and I am not going to use. He is the children's father and I was the only address he could use to get out of jail."

"Okay, okay," I said. "I am your friend here."

It was a shame, I understood the dilemma, same story different day. It was also amazing to me how the kids were used in their rationalization. Too bad they had not discussed their options earlier.

Annie's husband did get on the program and I got him assigned to me. I knew I might have a conflict of interest since I was Annie's counselor. So I cleared that agenda with him and then with her. They both stated they were glad I had been assigned to him.

I did not cut this poor guy much slack and indeed he was a slacker. I do not think he lasted on the program for more than two months. He was never clean and never held a job for more than two days. He became a no show, she must have stopped paying the methadone bill and to me that was a good sign. I choose to believe that Annie was strong enough to hold her boundary line, I never saw either one of them again.

~ ~ ~

Simon came into the parking lot in a clean Mercedes Benz donned with a fedora hat and two women in the car by his side. His smile shone broadly, I could see it from the window. He had a bounce to his step. He was a sharp-dressed man and he actually opened the doors for his ladies which appeared to be clients about thirty years younger than him. This was not really strange, pay the methadone bill or have good drugs, no flattery needed. They were just doing what they had to, right?

Simon was signing onto the program when Ethel announced to me, "You have a new intake."

I had so much fun with this man, he had such a joyful attitude and appeared to have a good heart both physically and soulfully. Simon proudly stated he was sixty-nine years old and just got out of prison, with no parole. He became involved with drugs during the Korean War and claimed to have provided the drugs to officers to supplement his Army pay. He said he had fourteen children to support and the extra money he made dealing really helped at the time. "Hey, it's a good thing I was locked-up for thirty years, who knows how many children I would have had!" he added.

Simon related that he got into trouble trying to continue the drug dealing when he was discharged from the service. He gave me a story about his last arrest that was somewhere between an Eliot Ness movie and the showdown at the OK Corral. He did not like to use drugs but did sometimes. He admitted his weakness was good-looking women and added it was a good thing I was taken. The other weakness was he did like to have a good time, "You know, a good steak dinner and a few cocktails."

Someone had been banking money for him while incarcerated because he received an inheritance of many properties in the area, all collecting rent payments and mortgage free. Simon was ripe for the women in the area, and sorry, but he would have made a perfect sugar-daddy for anyone! We had a good laugh for the first few sessions. I told him things had changed since he got out and to be sure to wear his *helmet* or *jacket* when he had a good time. Like a sixteen-year-old boy with hormones raging, this man was in my office every Friday for a box of protection.

One day he got real serious and asked about a girl he had met. Simon told me, "She is sick and needs care." He answered my round of questions: "Yes, she is someone he met on the street" "Yes, she is addicted to heroin" "Yes, I guess you are right, I don't need to rescue anyone."

Simon was good friends with the twins, Bert and Ben. It was the geriatric club. Six or seven of these guys hung-out at Ben's place. Ben had learned to cut hair in prison so they all hung-out at his house during the day, of course, the local women seemed to show up there too.

I had Bert and Ben on my caseload, it took me a long time to get their names straight but it became easier after the first few weeks. Bert was a mess and Ben had it together. These guys were in their seventies. One of my younger female clients filled me in on the gossip about Ben's place. I discovered this was just one of the problems around methadone clinics. If you want to find someone to be *naughty* with it was easy, just a different sort of social club.

Simon started to enjoy those steak dinners a little too often and got a ticket for driving under the influence, alcohol he told me. His attitude changed and he started using heroin, shortly after this he was back in prison. He knew when he was going and we started the dose taper. He wrote me once, it was a "thank you" letter. The men who have spent time in prison have such nice handwriting.

Ben and Bert were total opposites, as I stated. Bert was the one I took to the doctor regularly, he was a mess. He did not bathe, used everything he could find or buy, and was usually drunk to-boot! Ben was always angry with Bert. Bert was weak and prey for some of the women clients; they used him, encouraged him, and hurt him. Ben was cool, short tempered, never anything much to say. He was low profile and I left him alone. Bert on the other hand was death waiting to happen.

Bert got in trouble one day over the ugliest working girl I had ever seen. She was twice as big as him, and I am sorry, just "butt-ugly" as my client's would say. Jack had to hide his eyes when she came to the clinic but I guess love knows no boundaries. Ben had tried to fight for his brother's affection and there were rumors he put a hit out on Bert's love interest. This was one of the saddest situations, nothing ever happened but the counselors were on alert. It all died down after a while, it was just such a helpless feeling.

In my opinion, there was no way one could effect change in Bert. I tried to talk to Ben but it was useless, he had taken care of his brother for years. Ben had a room at his place for Bert and if he left everybody alone, he could continue to stay there. But Bert continued to use; continued to dose; and continued to not bathe unless there was a baptism, funeral, or birthday party. He was the first client that I raised the dose to 100 milligrams when we received permission to go that high. The only effect was more chemicals in his system, he admitted to not using for a whole two or three days.

Carlos was also a member of the geriatric group, in fact, he just had major by-pass surgery when he transferred to the clinic. He had a heart attack at his favorite restaurant, Burger Heaven. He loved their croissant breakfast. Bert and Ben found Carlos slumped-over his favorite booth and took him to the hospital. It was harder for me to get him to give up those breakfasts than the heroin!

Carlos lived alone in a room. He said the two joys in his life were eating at Burger Heaven and his appointments with me. Such flirts these older guys were! Carlos was always fearful of missing his ride to or from the clinic. Ben would not wait for those he gave rides to, he did not want to be indisposed in any way. Nice old men, nowhere to go, nothing to do, and much too easy for trouble to find them.

~ ~ ~

As you look at our youth today in their costumes of baggy pants with under-wear showing or cutoffs and long white socks with slippers, sometimes it is hard not to laugh. One has to remember what we wore at their age. What is really sad is when you see fifty-five-year-old men in these outfits! Cardo was on my caseload for over three years, he could not remember my name but told his social workers to ask for "the lady in black." My thinking is when you get up early and get dressed in the dark, if you wear black you always match.

The first time I met Cardo he was on his bike with his headphones on. He was bald, had no teeth, and was related to almost everyone coming to the clinic. Cardo was not evil anymore, just naughty. He was always getting into trouble, it was more like babysitting. He was too old for the younger clients and too young for the geriatric club.

There were several in his age group though and these were the ones we needed to handhold. They would hang around the clinic mostly because they did not have anywhere to go and nothing to do. This group of clients was physically and so-cially impaired and could not work. They had previously abandoned their families for drugs and prison and now their children and wives did the same to them. When they were clean they were kind, remorseful, and so very lonely.

I tried to incorporate these guys into some of the local youth organizations that help keep kids off the street and off drugs, but they were not welcome. Each rejection they received just validated to them that they were useless drug addicts. So they would return to do what they did best, loiter around the clinic premises.

Our responsibilities at the clinic include taking action to get keep clients out of the parking lot, so after Moses asked them once or twice to leave with no response, a counselor would be called to get control of their client. It was like catching a thirteen-year-old sneaking a cigarette but these were fifty plus year-old men with serious criminal backgrounds selling their prescription drugs, or whatever they found that day to sell.

One day, I caught two of my clients. I came around the corner just at the right time to see the actual exchange, two hands outreached. Cardo started with, "Uh, he was paying me back money he owed."

Ivan smiled, as did Cardo, because they knew I was not stupid and that I knew they knew this. I had a hard time not smiling myself.

"Yeah," I replied, "and I was born at night but not last night. Get the hell out of here right now before I go medieval."

The next week when I got called down to the parking lot again, I had to get more than serious. I started out, "Look kids, we got a real problem. This is a residential neighborhood, people do not like drug dealing where they live. This is a drug treatment

facility and whether or not you are dealing drugs is not the issue, if they think you are, then it must be. Get it?"

I continued my lecture, "If you want to get the clinic closed and go without methadone *and* leave me unemployed, keep it up. If not, go three blocks in any direction you want but get out of here or I will put you on contract. Don't play me for stupid, get out of here now or there will be a hold on your dose for contract signing tomorrow." This was all it took, usually.

Human beings have their own cycle of behavior. As I am training my puppy right now, I recognize that animal behavior is not all that different. These guys would back-off for a few months then do it all over again. For a time, I got so sick of the spiel that I took to closing my eyes, putting my fingers in my ears and loudly droned, "Lala la, hear no evil, see no evil, speak no evil. If you are out of my sight before I count to three, I will *perform* no evil."

The codeine and Valium was especially valuable on the street around fee detox time. It might be on the other side of the building or across the street but they knew who had it. I knew all it took was a little action and the dealing started all over again.

Cardo had a metal plate in his head and he needed pain medication in the winter. He always wore a knit cap but that did not help him much. I could not get his prescription cleared on a seasonal basis, so he would use his own drug of choice. For a while, Cardo was really getting it together. Physically I do not know how he did it, he was always getting hit by cars on his bike.

He started to follow one of my suggestions of getting on a different bus each day to explore the area. These adventures would not cost him a dime with his bus pass. He thought about it for a while and much to my surprise, he did it. For almost two weeks straight, he went to another city for the day.

Then I suggested he go to the beach, "It's so hot out and if I can't go, someone should!"

Well, Cardo had the best time going to the beach three days in a row. Like a kid, he could not wait to share the excitement of his adventures. Then when he had not reported his adventures for an entire week I asked him, "Where are we going today, Cardo?"

With sadness he said, "Just home."

"What? The great adventurer lost his spirit?"

He said so very sadly, "It's no fun alone and I can't get nobody to go with me." We were supposed to discourage the clients from socializing but here I had a group of guys that needed to do *anything*. My inner logic told me *What is the worst that can happen? They get high together in a different city, big deal.* So, I tried my best to enroll the others into the "Adventure Spirit Class." No success I am sorry to say.

One day Cardo was going to be evicted from his room and we needed to find him shelter. As it turned out, his doctor placed him and another of my clients in an assisted living facility. Of course, this facility's staff had no idea that these guys were on methadone. I knew this facility personally, scary as it was, because my mother had stayed there.

Have you ever been to a board and care, or what they now call assisted living? Not one that I have ever visited smelled good, looked nice, or the people living there actually seemed grateful to be alive. But when I heard where they were, I was glad. I thought *Hey, this is great, especially since my Mom is not there anymore.*

I encouraged them to get out and socialize, go to the organized events, do something! On one of his outings, Cardo bought some paper and pencils. When he came in, he proudly displayed his work to me. I discovered he liked to draw but he could not afford to buy materials so I brought in some old stuff my daughters did not use. I figured I would encourage Cardo's artistic talent, right? It worked for a while and sparked some enthusiasm.

Cardo continued having a good time flirting, laughing, drawing, and going places. He was clean and complying with his medications. Well, he must have had too much fun because he was kicked-out of the home! Cardo claimed they told him he was too healthy to stay there but he was not healthy for long. He had another bike accident and was hospitalized for a long time.

12 | Sometimes Compassion Works

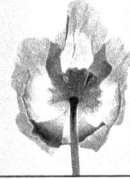

Jack warned me about Chewy before I met him. He said he was the meanest, orneriest, strongest guy he had ever met and that he was still alive was a mystery of science. Chewy was angry at everyone and about everything, he did not have one nice thing to say. This day was introduction day for Chewy. Jack suggested that I establish my authority right at the beginning and to remember, "Most bears that growl have thorns in their paws."

When Chewy arrived, he got out of the medical bus and fell, so started the language, "Goddamn it, son-of-a-bitch. Shit, somebody goddamn help me get up for Christ's sake."

Since I witnessed the whole thing while waiting for him, I was right there and I grabbed his cane and his hand. He was about four feet ten and maybe a hundred pounds. He still had on his robe from the hospital and seemed embarrassed. What a way to begin our relationship. On top of that, I got to be the one to ask him for a urine sample!

I helped seat Chewy who was obviously frazzled, weak, and angry at life. He was getting his papers out mumbling mostly swear words when I said, "My name is Allie. I am your counselor."

"Oh shit, just get me my dose and get me the hell out of here now!" expelled from his mouth.

I said, "Look, Mr. Diego. I understand your situation and some of your pain, as well as, your frustration. But I will not allow you to talk to me like this or to treat me with such disrespect until, or if, I earn it. It is not my fault that you are sick, dependent on methadone, or miserable that you are still alive. I can be your friend or your enemy, your choice, but you are stuck with me and I am stuck with you. Do you understand what I just said?"

He nodded yes with his head down and did not look up.

So I said, "If you will excuse me, I will get the doctor to readmit you."

He nodded again.

The doctor was around the corner and heard the whole thing. He was laughing at me and said, "If he cannot urinate, I can wait until tomorrow to get the sample." I asked God to bless the doctor.

I returned to Chewy's reinstatement order and asked him if he could give me a urine sample now.

He repeated, "Now? goddamn... son-of-a-bitch."

"Stop that, a simple yes or no works for me," I said in my best stern mother's voice.

"No," he replied.

I said, "Okay, if you promise to watch your language and try to be my friend, I will ask the doctor if we can wait until tomorrow since you do not feel well and just fell."

"Okay," he agreed.

"Can you stand in line?" I asked.

"Yeeeeeeesss," he said with the most sarcastic yes I had heard all week.

I helped him get on the bus back to the board and care facility. Then he told me, "I need a take-home for the weekend." It was an order, not a request. "It's in my chart. Call my daughter, she will give the details. Thank you and good-bye."

Well, at least he said thank you! I looked the driver in the eyes and thanked him for waiting because he did not have to. I smiled and thought *Chewy and I are making progress.*

I called Chewy's daughter in the afternoon and shock of all shocks, it became a counseling session. She vented her frustrations with her father's attitude and behavior. She indicated, and his charts confirmed, that he went to her home every weekend. She was doing her best. It is not that she did not want him to live with her but with her work, children, and his daily dosing of methadone this was the best she could do. I suggested that when she brought him next time, we could have a talk.

Normally, a take-home request needed a couple of days to be processed, but I started the paperwork right after I talked to his daughter. The doctor and I discussed Chewy's situation and decided to put him on a medical take-home just to keep him away from the clinic. He was clean, had serious medical conditions, and he fell almost every time he came to the clinic.

When Chewy and his daughter and granddaughter showed up, he was his usual cantankerous-self, but just a bit more controlled. I watched him from my office, he did not see me. It was amazing to see the love and appreciation of his granddaughter's assistance and she paid no attention to his harsh words. He went directly to the restroom and demanded a bottle *now*, like he was the only one at the clinic. *You just gotta love that about some people* I thought to myself.

"Hey, good morning Chewy. How are you today? Is this your granddaughter?" I asked.

"I don't have time for this. Do you want me to piss, goddamn it, or not?" he said in his cheery voice.

"Here you go," I said and gave him a bottle. "When you are done, we are going to chat for a minute."

"Goddamn, I don't have time for this business of yours, give me that damn bottle," he snorted.

"You can leave the bottle in the window and flush the attitude, okay Chewy?"

"Goddamn it," he complained with his cane pushing the door open then slamming it on the wall.

His granddaughter and daughter began to apologize, "I am sorry, he really is…"

I said, "It's okay, I know he doesn't mean it. I am going to have a talk with him and I don't know how it will turn out, but he likes to go to your house doesn't he?"

"I think so," the daughter said then added, "It's hard to tell sometimes."

"I have done him a big favor he doesn't know about yet. I will tell him a thing or two that just might help both of us, if you back me up." Shaking her head, she agreed.

Chewy came out of the restroom snarling, "Now what the hell did you want?"

I helped him to one of Doc's examining rooms and closed the door. I said, "Look, you need people to help you and how much help do you think you are going to get if you keep being an obnoxious, cursing, cranky, miserable-to-be-around person?" He put his head down and said, "I don't mean to be bad."

I said, "I know you don't feel good and it is a bitch to be old and broken, isn't it?"

"Yes," he said with his head down.

"Do you like getting out of the home and visiting with your daughter?"

"Yes."

"Would you go out of your way to put up with her if she treated *you* the way you treat her?"

"No."

"So why add to your misery? Try to *pretend* to be a nice person. Do you want to come here every day, or once a week?" I asked knowing the answer.

He looked up and said, "What the hell do you think?"

I said, "Talk nice and see what happens."

"Once a week," he nicely replied.

I said, "Okay, I am going to invite your daughter and granddaughter in here. If you say you are sorry for being mean and ornery and I get good reports on your behavior, I will arrange for you to come only once a week."

"Really?" he asked with a gleam in his eyes.

"Yes, and I also want you to be nice when you get here, like with a smile on your face once in a while." Then I added as an afterthought, "By the way, it would be really cool if you could watch your language. I don't mind so much but your granddaughter doesn't need to hear it."

"Okay," he agreed.

"I have the papers here, the doctor has signed them," I said as I held the paperwork in front of him.

"Really?" his eyes open wide this time.

"Yes," I confirmed.

"Nobody has done anything like this for me in a long time. I am sorry. I don't mean to be mean," he apologized again.

That is all it took. For a long while, I greeted the bus when he arrived, took his urine without incident, had some good chats, and his outlook improved a great deal. He then hooked-up with a babe from the home. They agreed to live in a cottage behind her daughter's house and were going to transfer to a clinic near them. Who would have ever guessed what a bit of compassion could do?

~ ~ ~

We had several clients on the program with diabetes. I really did not know much about the disease, other than the person needed to watch their diet and sometimes take medication. I had one client in particular which I thought his drug use might be related to his sugar level and I discussed this with him. He was constantly on fee detox, heroin was not his drug of choice, it was cocaine. He stated he used it when he took his medication for diabetes because he felt so sluggish afterward. I asked the doctor about this but he just rechecked the drug usage. Then I asked the other counselors but they were not interested.

This particular client was open with me so we talked about his mood swings, diet, and drug interactions. We concluded it was his sugar level that made him feel like he needed an "upper." There is actually sugar in methadone which he also did not need. This client's mood swings were like Javier and my husband's which I suspected was a reaction to their sugar intake. About this time, Javier and my husband's current behaviors were driving me crazy. What seemed funny to them one day was not the next; one minute they remembered things, the next minute they did not. It seemed as though I could not do anything right at home or at work!

~ ~ ~

A few months after I went to work at the clinic, my mother's health declined. She lived close to the clinic and at the time was staying in assisted living just a few blocks away. It worked out great, I went to visit her on my lunch hour almost every day. Sometimes, I would stop by after work or if I was going in that direction on the weekend. She did well until Christmas when her physician suddenly called the family in to make final arrangements for her. She had an episode three days before Christmas and was in the hospital again. Her doctor of the last fifteen years told us it was most likely the end.

My sister and I had laughed about our Mom and her survival, she had come close to death several times. We took so many phone calls of her imminent death that we became numb to the possibility. However, we had never received a call from the doctor like this one before, so we took it more seriously than just another Code Blue in the emergency room.

Javier had scheduled the clinic to close at noon for a Christmas Eve luncheon. It was no big deal, a pot luck. I stayed awhile then asked to be excused at 1:00PM for an appointment with the family and my mother's doctor. I explained she was terminal but Javier did not understand why it could not wait until after the party. When we arrived, much to our surprise, Mom had a rebound. She even had a temper tantrum on New Year's Eve because she wanted to leave to celebrate!

When my sister and I went to visit her we had to tell her, "Sorry, the doctor says you must stay here for now and then go back to assisted living."

She said, "Over my dead body!"

We both said, "Maybe."

Then I said, "You are on borrowed time, don't push it, Mom." She was upset and we were upsetting her more, so we left.

Mom kept a phone number she had written down from one of those grocery store bulletin boards. The person advertising offered to run errands and do housekeeping. Mom called the number right after my sister and I left the hospital. She offered the lady one hundred dollars to come pick her up from the hospital and take her home! She wanted to make two stops on the way, the assisted living home to get her belongings and the market. Of course, the woman jumped on it.

After Mom returned home, I went to visit her after work twice a week. We went to dinner, Wal-Mart, K-Mart, and the grocery store. I was her only escape. At this point, my sister had had it with her and was called for emergency situations only. Our brother was the smart one, he moved out-of-state years ago when our father died. Mom and he were still close, however, and he received a daily phone call from her.

One day when Javier was looking for me at lunch, everyone told him that I went to visit my mother at the hospital. I actually had returned early and was eating lunch when he came in. He said in a sarcastic tone, "Gee Allie, I thought your Mom was supposed to be dying last Christmas."

I said, "She was and is, what's your point?"

I do not think he ever believed I was at the doctor's on Christmas Eve stressing over her arrangements with my family. I felt not an ounce of compassion.

~ ~ ~

One of the counselors, Lupe, had been at the clinic for over one year when I was hired. She was all of five feet tall and just twenty-two years old. She did not have a driver's license or her citizenship either, but she was bilingual. As a group, we helped her with the driver's test, citizenship, résumé, and threw in suggestions that she indeed should get back into school to get certified.

Lupe had a hard time with the clients. Most of them would not accept her as a counselor simply due to her age. They commented it was like getting a lecture from one of their children. She had learned about life and the field of addiction but wanted to get additional credentials. Lupe was a good counselor, just young. She had applied to various graduate programs and desperately needed a letter from Javier for entry.

We had fun observing Lupe and her air-freshener fights which she would get into with Jack. Lupe hated the smell of green apple and Jack's office was right next to hers. One day, he found a crack in the wall where he could use a straw-like device to spray her office with the green apple scent. So in retaliation, Lupe would toss shredded papers in his office. We never knew when we would hear, "I hate that smell" or "Don't throw that shit in here!" It was the little things that helped us stay sane. When Javier refused to type the letter she needed, it was not long before Lupe left us, then came her replacement.

There were no interviews for Lupe's replacement, Jody simply appeared from nowhere, almost the next day. She looked like trouble from the moment I met her. Due to Javier's work ethic if you recommended someone, they usually got the job. Jody's recommendation was from an unknown resource. She was tall, Hispanic, and I sensed, using something.

Lupe, Angie, Black Todd, Davey, and Javier were the youngest counselors at the clinic, in that order. The rest of us were in the you-should-know-better age group. Jody showed up in a low-cut blouse that was of a see-through material, a very short skirt, and very high heels. She was young and looking for trouble, she found it. All but Black Todd and Joe were in shock over the fact that Javier actually hired Jody. The buzz of conversation regarding Jody did not stop from day one. Joe took her under his wing quickly, there appeared to be some competition from Black Todd, but he was already in trouble with the religion thing.

Everything was annoying about this girl. When she used the computer, you could hear her pound the keyboard throughout the building. She also flirted shamelessly with the clients. She had worked at a clinic previously but claimed to need a tremendous amount of training and spent lots of time with Joe. Her office was at the opposite end of the building, next to Javier's. So she always had to use my exit which meant I had to endure her loud high heel steps from her office to mine. Of course, Joe's office was in the middle. You would think someone would have gotten the hint that something was not right when Jody slipped on the stairs the second week on the job and threatened to file a claim. No one stepped up to suggest any misconduct on her part.

Joe got his job through Jack. They had been friends for years, meeting at AA and helping each other with their sobriety. Jack was close to Joe's wife, children, and grandchildren. Jack knew the behavior between Jody and Joe was a sign of trouble and was fearful of what might come of it. People can be stupid when it comes to believing that no one will notice the changes in their behavior or moods. It can be all too evident.

Joe had been at the clinic for over three years, sober for six. Jody was the same age as Joe's daughter who had a child the same age as Jody's child. The relationship started with Joe and Jody going to lunch together. After a while, we noticed they always ate their lunch *after* they returned. They were also in each other's office most of the day. With those high heels, I always knew where she was walking to or from.

Then the door slamming started. Also, Jody and Joe frequently talked to each other on the phone tying-up the intercom. So then we heard phone slamming too! Within three weeks of Jody's arrival, we noticed she had broken out with sores around her mouth. By the fifth week, Joe had them too. Soon, Joe's personality changed. It was easy to figure out what was going on between them. They were absent on the same days, they spent long periods of time in each other's office; and of course, the door slamming and door pounding was a big clue. It became difficult to ignore the grabbing-ass games in the file cabinet room, they were worse than teenagers. We just tried to ignore it all.

Then Joe's wife called and asked if we noticed anything different in Joe's behavior. At this point, the clients were now talking about them as the "clinic couple." Throughout all this drama, Jody's work and personality appeared stable. The clients knew what she was up to from day one. The pressure was on Javier, he had to do something.

It was bad enough that all of us had to deal with Jody and Joe's affair but it was also obvious that Joe had relapsed. He claimed his back pain had returned and he was taking codeine. *Hmmmm,* I wondered, *what made his back go out?*

The next thing we knew, Jody was gone and she was suing the clinic for sexual harassment. Poor Black Todd was also accused in the suit and was found guilty, he was let go. Needless to say, the affair ended, we think. It took Joe about three more months to lose his job due to his drinking. He made his choices. The clinic would have helped him but his shame got the best of him.

At the time, the census at the clinic was on a steady decline. We did not need to replace the two counselors right away. White Todd, my friend, was promoted to clinic manager. He would now have a reduced caseload and I was the one who was elected to train him. The clients were distributed between the rest of the counselors. I was assigned Mona's husband, Roberto.

13 | Sweet Success

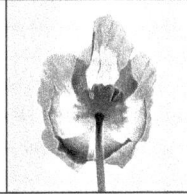

Roberto and his wife, Mona, had been on the program as Aretha would say, "Since Jesus was a baby." They were the best of clients, low profile and they rarely requested dose changes. If there was evidence of drug use, it appeared to have been casual use explained by an unreported prescription, not a daily thing. They had a daughter and she was obviously loved and cared for by both of them.

While I was out on leave, Mona had been transferred to another counselor which was a good thing, I think. I was not having any progress with all her medical problems. She was overweight, her diabetes was out of control, and her blood pressure was critical. She was an intelligent woman without the usual trail of children and husbands.

Mona had once obtained a really good job and claims her biggest regret was leaving it. This was when she fell into the life she knew but did not want. Most of our sessions were regarding Mona herself, her history and concerns about her daughter but nothing regarding her marriage or husband. So now I was to counsel Roberto. I put a message in for him to see me as soon as the dispensing nurse knew he had arrived.

I met Roberto at the stairs to advise him that I was now his counselor. I could see from the top of the stairs he had *attitude*. Wearing his bad boy costume of the knit cap pulled down to his eyes, dark sunglasses, baggy pants with knee-high white socks, and the damn slippers.

"Thanks for your time Roberto," I began. "I just wanted to let you know since Joe is gone, you have been assigned to me. If I can do anything for you, do let me know."

"Okay," he said, "you can leave me alone. I am a fucking drug addict and alcoholic and none of your lectures are going to change me. Okay?"

I replied, "Hey, what is this all about? I was your wife's counselor for almost a year, I don't think she had any complaints."

He said, "We don't talk about what goes on here when we're at home. All I know is every time Joe called me up to his office, he would go on and on about what a piece of shit I am. I usually felt so bad after that I would go score, or just buy a bottle."

"I don't do that, not my style. If you use, it is your choice. I am not going to knock my coworkers but I can tell you that Joe was in recovery himself. He achieved sobriety through AA and NA, same as Jack. The difference between Jack, myself, and Joe is that Jack and I went to school, we were trained to do this work." I now had his attention and the sunglasses came off.

"Really?" he asked.

I continued to tell him that I thought all humans were born to be addicted in some way. As he lit his cigarette, I knew the wall between us had been broken so I continued, "Have you ever noticed how people always park their cars in the same place or eat the same food?"

He said, "Yeah, I do that."

"There you go," I confirmed. "Where do you go for food?"

"Burger Heaven," he says, "so like you have a problem with hamburgers too?"

"This is serious," I said.

He laughed.

I continued, "Usually there is something behind the addiction, something that hurts and you learned that the way to avoid the pain is to get rid of it by drinking, using, or medicating."

"That makes sense," he replied.

"My thing is to figure out what hurts, deal with that and find a different way for you to respond or be. All you know is what you know but maybe I know something else. So can we give it a try?"

"You're not going to force me to go to a meeting?" he asked.

"I can't force you to do a damn thing you don't want to do. In fact, I forbid you to go to any meetings, okay?" I laughed this time and he laughed too.

I asked him if he was using and he said, "Sometimes, not often."

"Do you want to stop?"

He answered, "Yes."

"Great, then you are halfway there!" I cheered.

"When do I get to see you again? I'll come tomorrow and we will start okay?" he asked with a hint of excitement.

"We already did!" I told him. He stood and gave me a hug and walked away smiling.

My first session with Roberto began with his apology for his attitude the first time we met. He explained he was just not going to go through what he did with the other counselor. That counselor (Joe) was the only one he had experienced at the clinic and he thought we were all the same. This was the reason he never requested a transfer to a different one. He then asked me for a 10 milligram dose increase.

I said, "No problem." He was confused as to why I did not make a big deal about it. I told him, "Why would I challenge a good thing. This tells me you have put some thought into the program and that you have quit being a heroin addict."

He smiled, took a sip of coffee and said, "This is good."

"Oh, one other thing. Again, this is your choice but alcohol will affect the methadone and ninety percent of the people that use needles for their drugs have Hepatitis C. So, if you want to encourage the disease that there is no cure for, continue drinking. Now, tell me about your childhood."

As I put my feet up on my desk and smiled, he sat back in his chair and did the same. We began a two-hour session where the man cried on two occasions and stated he had not cried in years. I swear all I said during that entire time was, "Go on, tell me more. "

Roberto was in my office once a week for one to two hours, whatever he needed he got. The change was immediate. The costume was gone. He had pride in his appearance, he did the best he could with his limited resources. Each change was noticed and praised, not just by me but by all the staff at the clinic. They were all aware of the counseling time he was putting in. First the long baggy pants were replaced, then the slippers were traded for new tennis shoes. He got haircuts on a regular basis and actually started exercising. I had explained to him the effects exercise had on serotonin levels in the body and the changes which occur. Also, just the pride he could own in doing something positive for himself.

The dose taper began and the changes became even more obvious. He got a job! The day he came to the clinic in a white shirt and tie, pressed dress slacks, hard shoes, and a suit coat, the staff rallied him. He had gone from gang-banger using, drinking, and on 80 milligrams of methadone to a productive taxpaying citizen on 5 milligrams with a target date to be methadone free!

It did take time for all of this to happen, mostly due to the fear and reality of the physical changes which happen with a reduced dose. Like anything else, it was his determination, constant reinforcement, and most of all, his immediate recognition of his own achievements which fueled him past the pain. Also, his success stemmed from identifying his past and present pain and working through it. In order to fix something, first it needs to be acknowledged.

Later, we had to slow the taper, detoxing usually gets worse toward the end. Roberto came down pretty fast and the anxiety, as well as, the physical symptoms of withdrawal were taking their toll on him. He agreed that the exercise helped and the spa eased his aching bones. I had also told him how to get free passes to health clubs and the socializing did not hurt either.

Now there were several problems that had to be addressed in his marriage and the pressure at home was growing beyond tolerable. This situation happens in dependent relationships. The dynamics of two sick people in a relationship works, but with one in recovery and the other still using, it falls apart.

Roberto no longer wanted drugs or drug users around his house. Since most of his wife's family used drugs, including his wife due to the stress of his transformation, he felt he was living in hell. My focus was to get Roberto off methadone and for him to move out of the neighborhood, out of the jungle. I used his daughter as an example every chance I could, "She is bright and beautiful, do you want her to end-up on a program?" I explained about the power of influence and how many times we seem to turn into our parents, even if we do not want to.

One day he came to me and said his son from a previous marriage had called him and had serious problems. The boy was twenty-three and in trouble with alcoholism and adultery. Roberto told me this was the exact age when his life went to heroin. Oh the pain of reality! He said everything I had told him about turning into our parents was true and he had to get his daughter out of the neighborhood. He was very concerned about taking her away from her mother but did not want her to end up like him or his son.

Another underlying fear and question Roberto had was could he still see me for sessions if he was off the program. He needed to hear that I would be available to him, I gave him that reassurance. He also learned to trust Jack and I told him that one of us would always be ready to help.

The last day came, Roberto swallowed his last dose of methadone. I printed a certificate for him to keep. We also bought him a cake and had a party at 5:30 in the morning! I had done the impossible, no, *Roberto* had done the impossible. But could he sustain it?

~ ~ ~

Mom had continued to use the lady who helped her escape from the hospital. Her name was Donna, that was the extent of my knowledge about her. I went to visit her after work one day and the remains of what appeared to have been a small party were scattered over Mom's kitchen, living and dining rooms.

Her front bathroom was completely torn apart. I asked her, "What is going on? It looks like the party got rowdy in the bathroom!"

She said, "There was a problem with the plumbing and Donna's boyfriend is a handyman so he came over with a friend to help. Don't worry, they will be back tomorrow to finish the job and I can use the back bathroom."

"Mom, what do you know about these people? There are lots of not-so-nice people out there," I said trying to get more information.

She said, "Don't worry, where do you think you got your judge of character skills from?"

"My father," I replied. She laughed. "No, really. I bet you guys partied together all night. You fed them and you paid for all of it, right?"

"Well, they had to eat. They had been drinking and working on the toilet until 11:00PM"

"Those are not normal working hours Mom and you have no business drinking," I scolded.

"But it was fun, damn it, and I hadn't had company in a long time, besides you that is, no offense."

Out of my mouth came, "How do you know that they are not on the program, uh?" Do not ask me why, but Donna never seemed to come around to "work" when I was visiting Mom.

Then one day soon after the party incident as Mom and I were driving into the mobile home park, she pointed out Donna's car. It looked uncomfortably familiar. Do not misunderstand me, there were a few girls on the program that I thought *could* work for my Mom, but I did not know this lady. So like an eagle, I am looking for this car the next day at the clinic and who do you think pulls up and is on the program? Right, Donna.

I do not think when the government set up the program to give individuals on general relief or Welfare training to become nursing assistants, that they realized they were helping set up one of the greatest senior citizen rip-offs around. My Mom was a prime target. She was spacey, disorganized, and left her credit cards, checks, and money laying all over the place. The worst of it was that people like my Mom were very trusting. She even gave Donna her ATM card and password on many occasions to get the cash necessary to pay her or to go to the market for her!

I talked to Donna's counselor and tried to get as much information as I could. She, of course, did not have much to say. I pulled up Donna's dosing history on the computer and got all the information I needed to know, she was dirty and using methamphetamines. Now mind you, Donna was Mom's hero, she saved her from the hospital and the assisted living facility. Donna also had a man-friend that might someday fix her toilet! Besides, she was fun company for Mom—bad company was better than no company for this lonely lady.

I waited for the next day after Donna dosed and stopped her in the hall. "Your name is Donna. It's a small world isn't it? I hear you are my Mother's right arm," I said trying to sound friendly.

"Oh, you are Allie and this is the clinic you work at?" she asked.

I said, "Yeah, coincidence, isn't it?"

Well, I did not have to say much and legally I could not. In a short time, Donna's truth came out. She was also working for a man, another senior citizen. She was caught using his credit cards to withdraw cash and had also sold his car. His family apparently lived out-of-state and had no clue until they came up for their quarterly visit, then all was discovered and the police were contacted.

Donna's boyfriend came by to ask Mom if she had money for Donna's bail, but for she said no this time. I think it was just too much for her and she was angry because it had been three weeks and her toilet still was not reattached. This was Donna's third strike and she would not be around again for a long while.

~ ~ ~

Ray was a nice man, he was not on my caseload yet but he was a good client. He was easy to spot, there were only two African-Americans on the program. Ray would standout anywhere. He was immaculate and had the build of an athlete. He was about six feet four inches in height and solid muscle. Ray worked, was clean, and always paid his bill on time. The car he drove was one of those great big Lincoln Continentals, it was immaculate too but it was always breaking down. This frequently occurred with many of the cars in our parking lot. It was also not unusual to witness police activity in the parking lot. We would all gather at the windows and watch from afar when they were present and/or an incident was taking place. This was one of those days.

There was always entertainment to be had looking out the windows at the clinic, the parking lot was as much fun as an "E" ticket ride at Disneyland™! Watching the clients come and go provided a good distraction for the stressed out counselors. It was hot, almost 12:20PM and rush hour for the clients. They were afraid of the clinic closing too soon, so most of the driving at this time of day was very erratic.

It was a tough call for this one client leaving the parking lot, we watched and agreed the officer appeared to have set her up. It looked like he stopped to let her make a left turn out of the lot and he was going to turn in, but he stopped her as their cars were parallel. He stated that she pulled out in front of him. The police car was blocking the driveway in the middle of the street and her car was on the other side. The officer called for backup, the woman with her purse spilled-out on the hood of her car was spread and cuffed while he searched her body. I saw no need for this, I felt it was harassment.

Not often, but on occasions like this, some officer would come around and pick on a client. Another time a man was sitting on the front stairs with his daughter, we were closed and he was waiting for his ride. The officers ran a check on him and the next thing you know there was a swarm of police cars and the man left in cuffs. His little girl was taken away. Just about anyone here could get arrested for something.

Ray's car had no reverse and where it had broken down he could have gotten out of the lot moving forward, if the officer had not blocked the driveway. Most of the clients would wait, not wanting to be harassed, but Ray had nothing to fear except being late for work. He was pushing the car backward when the brakes went out and his car rolled right into the police car! I hoped that cop spent the next two days filling out forms because it was truly an accident. No problems for Ray this time, thank goodness, and the lady was let go too.

Johnny was one of the main reasons that no staff members parked in the clinic parking lot. Johnny was in his late sixties, nearly blind, senile, and using, as well as, on methadone. His car did not have an inch on it that was not dented, he even has a huge Band-Aid™ sticker on it about three feet long in one place. Just watching him come and go was entertainment enough for the day, as long as *your* car was not parked in the lot!

One day we were going to celebrate a staff's birthday, which we did often. These parties were planned in advance so we could close the clinic for half an hour early and meet at a nearby restaurant. We had all left the building except for Angie; she was bringing the cake which she hid in her office. It was a bit scary at the clinic sometimes. We really had no real security and sometimes clients would come up the stairs unannounced, or someone would come just to look around for an HIV test or something.

Well, Angie came out of her office with the cake in her arms and a man was standing there in the hall. She screamed at him and they both almost had heart attacks. He explained that he was the architect from San Diego who was suppose to inspect the building for proposed changes.

After gaining his composure he asked, "What type of medical center is this again?"

Angie explained that we were closed until 11:00AM and that if he wanted to follow her to the restaurant, he was welcome. She felt she owed him something since she scared him half-to-death. He followed her to the restaurant and joined us, we all had a good laugh.

When we returned, the architect parked in the lot. We were still in the social mode and looking out the window when Bonnie exclaimed, "Didn't anyone tell that guy about the parking lot?"

Just then Johnny pulled up. We all started laughing about the what-ifs and the poor man's introduction to the clinic when it happened. We watched and shouted in unison, "Oh no, no, stop!"

It really was not funny but at least it was a rental car. This was why you never ever park in the parking lot at our clinic. Remember, it is the little things one must know around a methadone clinic to survive.

14 | Struggling with Karen and Myself

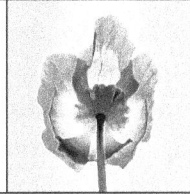

I discovered I had gained thirty-five pounds and was sleeping way too much. I could not catch up on my bills, they were not going away. I had no social life to speak of and I was crying constantly. The job no longer seemed fun, life was no longer fun. I went to see my doctor. Have you ever seen the cartoon that says, "I can't prescribe antidepressants for you, you have good reason to be depressed!" Well, that was what the doctor pretty much told me.

My doctor also asked, "What's going on in your life? Last year, you were in perfect health. You appear to have stress-induced asthma and high blood pressure. You have gained thirty-five pounds, look like hell, and you have a hernia."

"A what...?" I asked.

She suggested the weight gain, stress, and maybe the hysterectomy two years earlier all had something to do with my condition.

"Do you want some time off?" she asked as she started writing down instructions for my hernia surgery.

The next day, I went to work and told the office that I was scheduled for surgery on Monday and would be taking some time off. My job was protected, I had two weeks sick leave accumulated and I thought I might be entitled to disability. No one at the clinic was surprised about my needing time off except for Javier. He actually did not return to the clinic until after my surgery.

I took off the full eight weeks, I was in pain for most of it but the sleep I got helped immensely. I thought about looking for some other kind of work but I was in no condition at the time. All the staff and the clients knew what I had been going through in my personal life and no one even expected my return, including me.

My husband admitted to being diagnosed with diabetes several months earlier. He finally decided to tell me and assured me it was under control. I watched him and Javier and was convinced now that all the conflict we had experienced was not me, it was them and their diabetic mood swings. It felt good at that time to trust my intuition again even though that did little for my marital tribulations.

Later during our gossip hours, we all laughed at who was more surprised at my return, the staff or me. I believe they all knew how honest I had been about not returning to the clinic after my medical leave. We were all in the same situation, counseling at the clinic was a hard job. The emotional factors alone were stressful, maybe that was why we had such great benefits and so much paid time off, no questions asked. Where else could I have a job with full medical and dental coverage, paid three weeks' vacation, and thirteen paid holidays? The clinic staff just needed to keep their clients low profile, not upset the doctor or the dispensing nurse, get great audits, and comply with state and federal regulations. It felt good to be missed while I was away, but it felt better to be a part of the team again.

The episode with Linda and Javier and all their erratic behavior pulled us together somehow. We were now more like a family than a group of people who worked together. Major changes were coming to the clinic. We did not have a clue how we were going to accomplish the new requirements of the additional counseling that would change from thirty minutes per month to fifty minutes per week.

There were also changes in our medical department. We now were to provide medical treatment to the indigent population or those who claim unable to pay for medical treatment. That meant medical care regardless of the Mercedes Benz they drove up in, their current designer clothes, or the showy diamonds. If they said they could not afford medical treatment, they got it for free at our clinic.

This new protocol created many new problems. First of all, the traffic around the clinic was unbelievable. Where were all these people supposed to wait? We now had two sets of budgets, two sets of census requirements, and the doctor was cranky to-boot. Trying to keep the clients straight, the loitering straight, and those waiting for treatment apart from those who just dosed was a riot.

One day, Doc was really frazzled and I had a bottle of Saint John's Wart with me. St. John's Wart is an herbal remedy for anxiety and stress. I went to the dispensing nurse and told her to tell Doc to pop a few of the St. John's pills but she said, "No, you do it."

I told her that I was not qualified to dispense and she was, so take a chance! She found her moment and presented the bottle to Doc with two tablets in hand. The next day, Doc asked me, "Allie, tell me about these pills."

I did and the following day Doc brought them to the staff meeting and told everybody to take one and for Javier to take two. Again, it was the little things that made my day.

~ ~ ~

Mom was being an unreasonable burden, I guess I would be too if I was her. She was housebound and in pain most of the time; she had her good days, but needed a reason to keep going. We kept pushing for her to move out-of-state. Financially, it would be better for her and she could spend time with my brother's children. They were the only little ones left and my niece was now being raised by a woman who was not her mother. No big deal, but it was enough motivation for my Mom to move. She left on my birthday; coincidence only if you did not know my mother.

I do not mean to sound disrespectful but it was hard being stuck in the middle between Mom, my daughters, my work, and my husband. I had one daughter in her second year of college and one daughter a senior in high school. I was Mom's only escape if she continued to live here and, do not forget, I lived with and worked for crazy men.

The move went great. My brother connected her to the Internet and I could write her every day. She emailed me updates on the daughter-in-law from hell. In January, two months after Mom moved, my husband and I separated and I had peace. Javier was at the office less and I felt good for the first time in two years. It was so obvious, it only took about a week when my daughter remarked, "You are glowing!"

On the other hand, my debts were three times my income and I could not comprehend how I was going to make it financially without my husband's help. But there was no way I would ask him so I had to plan my survival. My credit had always been solid gold, in fact, that was part of how I got into this financial mess. I had funded my business, the Holistic Health Center and paid tuition for both the girls before going to work for the clinic. My job did not pay too well, and I had not made a dent in my debts.

I knew it would take at least six months before the foreclosure of our house and I had enough equity to pay off the debt, if the house sold. My youngest would be out of school in April, so I was not worried about a roof over her head. We could eat and have lights and heat until the house sold, or she graduated. I soon was able to sleep again and I started working out to gain strength and endurance. I had not heard one word from my husband and that was just great with me.

Javier dished out some flippant remark about how the "super-counselor" would take care of the additional counseling now required of us. I replied that I already spent the newly required time with my clients, now I would have the opportunity to document it without making anyone look inadequate.

"Seriously Javier," I added, "have you ever thought about having yourself tested for diabetes? Did you know it is at epidemic levels for Hispanics? In fact, you know my husband and I just separated, well I think that is why we fought so much."

"Really?" he said with interest.

Evidently, I finally touched his soul. He sat down in my office and the *nice* Javier was back. I described to him what I had witnessed in my husband and my client's behavior.

He shared some of what he was going through and said, "You really are a good counselor aren't you?"

I could not tell if he was being real with that remark or just smart-mouthing again, but he went down to the doctor's office and had his sugar level tested! Gee whiz, guess what? Yep, it was high.

The staff at the clinic rallied me the queen of confrontation. I told them, "I have worked with murders, carjackers, and thieves. So what's to fear with Javier?"

Now when the boss walks around and acts like a jerk, the standard comeback is, "Excuse me boss, but have you followed your diet today? Like, what is your sugar level today?" Power, I love it.

~ ~ ~

"Oh, honey, looks like we are really having a bad hair day aren't we?" a voice came from nowhere. As I turned around there stood a queen, not a regular sight at the clinic. Most of the gays in this area were not so colorful.

I said, "I beg your pardon?"

He said, "It must be the weather but maybe we should consider some color?"

I said, "I don't think we have met yet, are you new?"

He related that he had just gotten on the program yesterday, "Thank God, my habit is breaking me. The dope just isn't worth it anymore, *ces la vie* to the party life. By the way, what do you think of my new pants? I know my ass is sagging but aside from that, do you think white pants work for me?"

I responded with a smile, "In those pants you should consider some hip-lifts if you want to draw so much attention to your ass."

He laughed and said, "Paybacks, uh?" Then seriously he said, "A little red would bring out your natural coloring. My name is Bobbie, with an 'i-e'. Can you please ring up my counselor?"

Bobbie, with an i-e, stood-out at our clinic no matter what he wore. There just were not that many men who wore eye shadow, if you know what I mean. His sister had been on the program and was pregnant and he came to help her with the new baby. It was a good thing, not only did Bobbie help us with our colors and keep us up to date with the latest free gifts at the makeup counter, but he turned out to be a great maternal influence with his new niece.

Bobbie came into the clinic one day and said, "Can you believe that cunt actually fell asleep at the park with this little angel, right after shooting up? Who knows what could have happened to her, of course, I called the authorities. Now I need letters from all of you here to help me get full custody of this little darling."

So what if his sexual orientation was something other than the norm; so what if he wore more makeup than I did; so what if his ass looked better in white pants than mine; and not many knew but, so what if he was HIV positive. He loved that baby and wanted to care for her. So, we each wrote the needed letters and Bobbie, with an i-e, became Mother of the Year at our clinic.

~ ~ ~

I was never really introduced to Karen, but I knew who she was. She was high profile just because of her looks. Even pregnant she had a great body, smooth coffee-colored skin, and deep green eyes. It was rumored she was gay, this would be her third child however. I knew the middle child, he came with her to the clinic while her daughter was in school. Karen lived with her mother who was on the program and much to my surprise, she was related to almost everyone at the clinic.

I had a male client who was boasting the impending birth of his new grandnephew. "Karen is my niece," he bragged. He told me the father of her children was insane and that he was real bad for Karen. "He is into rough sex, he almost killed her the last time he was out, thank God he is back in jail."

The clinic was its own little world. News traveled fast, often to my regret. One time, I wrote a letter for a client to get out of doing General Relief work for reasons other than were stated, but the client and I had our reason. Then I get called into the doctor's office and he instructs, "Javier has asked that all letters be signed either by me or himself, is that understood?"

I said, "No problem, what's up?"

"Well, while I was away on leave one of Angie's hard-to-handle clients wanted a letter written to get him out of General Relief work and she refused to do it stating that it was against clinic policy. She wanted this guy to get a job. Anyhow, the girl I wrote the letter for was the sister of the guy on Angie's caseload and he produced a copy of the letter I had written for her. Angie was pissed, so *ta da*, no more letters!"

It was a Thursday, the sunrise and morning were so beautiful I found more excuses than usual to wander around the clinic. As I looked over to the far side of the parking lot, I saw Karen and her mother. She looked and we made eye contact. Her expression said, "I need to talk to you, but I don't want to hear what you have to say." She looked different, the kind of different I did not want to hear about.

Karen continued to get her nearly three month old son out of the infant seat in the back and stood up with him in tow, "Oh, Hi Allie, I need to talk to you. My Mom thinks I'm pregnant."

I knew it! my brain was racing. I asked myself *What's the procedure? What's the right thing to say? "Oh shit" just won't do.*

Karen continued to talk while we went inside, "Maybe I'm just late, my period hasn't gotten right since the baby. Maybe we should test next month?"

"Karen, you know the game. I cannot wait; I have to test you now. There are some things I can forget and pretend I don't see, but not this," I tell her as I turn around and look in to her tear-filled eyes. I knew that she knew she was pregnant and the test would break her denial.

"Can I at least dose first?" she asked.

"Sure," I said "there is no rush." She handed me the baby and I added, "I know you won't leave without this!"

Her son was beautiful and so full of life. Some of the clinic babies are so still and small but not this guy. Karen came around the corner with a posture that stated *I hate my life but it's not your fault.* She said, "Where's the bottle?"

"It is in the window, all set for you," I told her.

I did not watch, I gave her some space. I thought this was the best approach, besides, it was a beautiful day and I was feeling good. She came out and said she left the sample in the window.

I asked her, "How did this happen? I thought Mike was still locked-up, I haven't seen him here in a while."

"He just got out five weeks ago, you know how it is..." she lingered. I knew.

Karen was one of the most beautiful girls at the clinic, Latina but no trace of gang membership. She could have been a model. She was born into a family of heroin users. Most of the clients were related in some way and they were all proud of their family members. The family connections were exposed to newcomers when there was a birth or death, the pride and the pain was right there.

Karen became my client through a case transfer right after her last baby was born. I knew her Mom. I had tested her before and she seemed to be a nice woman. At our first session, Karen told me her story like someone had pressed "Play" on a tape recorder.

"Ya see," she explains, "Mom used, my Dad was in prison and I remember these low-lifes always around the house. I kept begging my Mom to quit but she never listened. I decided I'll show her just what it's like to have someone you love use shit. So one day, I flirted with one of the guys that I always saw fixing at my house, he was a lot older, twenty to be exact. It was Mike. I thought this would get my Mom's attention. He gave me some the first time I asked and then the first time we did it, I got pregnant. My Mom swears if I look at a dick, I end up pregnant. She is right. After I had that baby, Mike got locked-up. It's a good thing because he is crazy. The last time he was out, baby number three came and I also had to testify against him. He got locked-up because of me."

"Karen, so like, why if you knew he was crazy and you didn't want to use again, why?" I asked her in frustration.

"He is my child's father, how could I say no?" she answered with sincerity.

I have never in my life witnessed such unconditional boundaries over and over as with our clients. "So, you are like five weeks along I take it? What happened this time, why did you see him?" I continued to ask questions wanting all the details.

"Oh hell, Allie, you know it's easier to give in than to fight. He would come over to the house at all hours pounding on my window. My Mom would get pissed and heck I needed a stroller for the baby. Welfare doesn't give you much, you know?"

"Ah, that explains all the bruises and such for the last month, right?"

"Yes," she said with her head down. "Look Allie, I gotta go, I'll see you tomorrow, okay?"

"Sure," I said as I gave the baby back to her.

I took the sample to the doctor and told him, "Most likely just a few weeks along." Then I arranged for her to see him tomorrow for the results.

"That is too bad," Doc stated. "Allie, what are we going to do with these people," he said more like a statement than a question. "Have you thought about going back to school? You would be a good doctor."

"Thanks Doc," I said, "but right now, I have a full plate."

Most of the time we counselors masked our feelings and personal opinions by complaining about the extra paperwork involved in our case management. We always tried to celebrate life and its possibilities, like how I always wore yellow on urine test day! Sick humor I told myself but someone had to remember to laugh, even if it was sick. I truly did not mind the urine testing most of the time, I got to see everyone. It was like catching up on the gossip at the corner store.

There really was no such thing as "surprise testing" unless there was a counselor change. Even then it was tough to stop the communication. The clients would run down the week without much effort. The users use, the cheaters cheat, and the clean ones go with the flow, pardon the pun. When a client decided to cleanup, he was anxious to prove it and hovered for the results, finally an opportunity for some pride. Perhaps a little different than a gold star on a spelling test, but the same effect.

The next day, Josie walked up and asked, "Testing again?"

"Yeah, time flies when you're having fun. Here is your bottle," I said and handed her a bottle.

I had already asked Jack if he could cover for me, I had a client that needed some special attention. Jack was the only one I could trust to not upset the clients and handle it without a major scene. I asked Josie if she could speed it up a bit because I saw Karen coming and Jack was on his way downstairs.

Being pregnant and on methadone was pretty serious stuff. The clients did not want you to know for sure they were pregnant because of all the clinic requirements. Heroin interferes with the menstrual cycle, so sometimes women did not know when they were pregnant. The period of indecision always arrived, reality versus fantasy. We actually insisted they go to an Obstetrician and get prenatal care which was not a simple task. Very few Ob/Gyns would take a high-risk methadone pregnancy.

Karen looked like she had been crying all night. She began, "Allie, I just feel so ashamed, I feel dirty. My Mom won't let up on me either."

"Well, Karen, we all make mistakes and sometimes we don't think things all the way through," I tried to reassure her.

Karen lowered her head, "The worst part is that Mike says it is not his."

"I don't mean to get personal Karen, but is it?" I asked.

"Christ Allie, I don't like men, you know that. He got out a few weeks ago, I feel so stupid."

"Well, some lessons are harder than others," I said trying to find something nice, not like her mother.

"I try not to get pregnant but when you're using you never know when your period comes and then MediCal won't let me tie my tubes because I am too young! Allie, answer me this, why don't they stop addicts from getting pregnant? I mean it's *my* body, right?"

I could not answer Karen's question, instead I told her, "Let's go back to see the doctor, quit beating yourself up. It takes too much energy to get down on yourself, besides 'it is what it is.' Look, the doctor will be here in just a second, I want you to have a really good weekend. Remember 'thoughts are things' so keep them positive."

Karen was staring at the floor and the tears were flowing. I held her shoulders and continued, "We are going to take three deep breaths. You don't want the doctor to see you crying, he will think I upset you." She started to smile so I added, "We are going to inhale the good and exhale the bad." We did three deep breaths together and she was laughing when the doctor walked in.

Sometimes there was just nowhere to dump all my feelings, thoughts, and the what-ifs. It was suppose to be just a job, right? Drawing the line between getting too personally involved or simply having normal human compassion was getting more difficult for me. Karen was born to a heroin-addicted mother. The influence of the drug programs in school and on television taught her that these people were "low-lives," however, they were also family members coming into her house on a daily basis. She said she remembered always giving her mother a hard time in an effort to change their lives. She did not go into detail but she must have been under a lot of pressure, more than most preteens at least. If you cannot beat them, join them, right? Karen finally gave up at age fifteen.

I called Planned Parenthood to get more up-to-date information. I was shocked and amazed at the problem confronting female methadone users. In my conversation with the representative, she stated that due to the laws and ensuing controversy it was a nightmare for them. Many of the choices for birth control were not even available to women like Karen due to MediCal, or a lack of money. They must wait thirty days for a tubal ligation after an abortion; and, for the women who respond to the offer, many are pregnant again within those thirty days!

There were also those who continued to get pregnant simply to maintain Welfare benefits. Many women would not take birth control pills because they did not have a regular cycle due to the methadone and, of course, the pill also made them feel funny or they worried about the medical complications. The counselors had a good laugh about that one! Clients would not hesitate to mix toilet water with their heroin but were afraid of headaches, blood clots, or bloating with the pill, go figure.

We always allowed our clients to make their own choices, we were not to influence them on this particular matter. Our clinic was lucky in a way because our doctor was compassionate. He was Hindu and did not comment on the pregnancies or the choice to abort.

"Well, Karen, the test results are back and you are pregnant," Doc reported.

"Oh, I knew it, so I have an appointment for tomorrow, I can't eat or drink anything before and they want me to dose right after. So, you think I can get a take-home?" Karen asked him matter-of-factly.

"I am sure that Allie will arrange that for you, won't you Allie?" Doc asked me.

"Sure, Doc," I told him as Karen and I left to go to my office. I told her, "Let me get the paperwork together. I need the phone number of the clinic you are going to use."

"Sure, here it is," she handed me a piece of paper with a phone number on it.

I made the call, "Doris? This is Allie at the Methadone Clinic, I spoke with you yesterday."

"Yes Allie, your client said you would be calling and I have a signed release," Doris reported.

"So do I and I am pretty sure of the documents you need so if you will give me your fax number, I will send them to you now," I told her.

Doris stated, "I wish I could say I have never done this before but I have. I wish I could do more for your clients but you know the system, the girls usually give up in all the bureaucracy. All we can do is try, right?"

"Thanks Doris, and thank you for arranging things to happen so quickly. Please send those flyers about your clinic too. I will put them in the lobby," I assured her.

Turning back to Karen I told her, "Well, Karen, here is your paperwork and take-home. I guess I'll see you on Monday."

I tried to reiterate all those reassuring statements like "Quit beating yourself up." "I think you are making the right choice." "Things will be okay." Nothing I said seemed genuine at that point.

~ ~ ~

As I returned to take over the testing of my caseload, Jack was complaining that this was winter and there was no reason he should be forced to look at clients in shorts during the months of November to April.

"Is there no justice in this world? Hey look," he said showing me the newspaper, "big bust in town, none of our clients involved though. I wonder what this will do to the price of stuff? Wonder if the census will go up?"

A couple of the clinic clowns came up to the window asking for a cup of coffee. Jack and I were the coffee junkies and usually enabled our clients. The coffee pot was empty and it was close to lunch so we offered to make a pot.

They said, "No, we want the good stuff you keep upstairs."

We had spoiled them. Like many at first, they thought coffee was coffee. They could not understand why Jack and I would make a trip once a week using money out-of-pocket to buy the good stuff. The only way we could relate the issue to them was tell them it was the difference between black tar and China white heroin, they got it.

Jack was the first one to signal me about anything around the clinic, the first one to check if I had a problem with anything, and the one to review my charts before case presentations. If he thought it would not fly, it would not fly. On the other hand, if I wanted it to fly, he could tell me how to make it into an eagle. He also was my biggest opponent (in the beginning) with my theories on addiction and recovery. Sometimes, he just plain pissed me off. He made me cry at one point and I did not talk to him for six months. He also taught me how to laugh after years of no laughter, and he reminded me that I was a woman. Jack became a good friend, and I love him.

Jack was what they called a 12 Step Nazi. He thought AA or NA was the only way because it worked for him. I have always been a holistic nut; body, mind, spirit stuff with lots of education and self-love, it is my motto. He laughed in my face many times and we had daily debates over it. His usual comeback was he had "been there, I had not." I had no argument with that, or so he thought in the beginning.

When I arrived, Jack was the only client-friendly counselor at the clinic. He was also the only other counselor who was certified, except for White Todd. Jack had completed his internship at our clinic and just never left. He understood addiction and the clients respected him for that. Jack was the man who claimed to have been stoned or drunk for most of his life and who also claimed to have destroyed most of his brain cells. He had more stories than anyone I have ever known. Believe me, we had plenty of opportunity to hear them. Half of his stories I could not help but wonder if they were true, but then I would look in the eyes and say, "I believe." The man did have an attitude, his was a self-proclaimed asshole and proud of it.

There is a common thread that you see in people who go through the recovery process. Their lack of self-love often shows up as anger. Jack could go from a compassionate person to a glowing red, foaming-at-the-mouth, angry bastard instantly. At those times, if it was not sarcasm, it did not come from his mouth. On the other hand, he evoked the kind of laughter that made you snort or wet your pants.

Political correctness did not exist at the clinic and between a few of us it ranked on the obscene. It was probably a coping mechanism. The counselors developed a very sick sense of humor when we were, as Jack would say, "Stuck on Ground Hog Day." Dealing daily, weekly, and monthly with the pain and suffering of our clients, we needed an outlet. I was the only one at the clinic who could get along with Jack on a regular basis. Do not get me wrong, we really were like family and truly did love each other, but Jack was like the asshole brother. Maybe it was one trait he learned growing up in an alcoholic household, as I did. Jack knew how to play the game. We learned how to stay one step *ahead* of the game of life. We learned the *Who's Who* directory and how to kiss ass to those who counted. We quickly learned the personality traits of those around us and how to *work* them.

I instinctively followed Jack's lead from my second day at the clinic. He knew I was using him as a mentor. It took him awhile before he trusted me. I would have to say our relationship started right after his fiftieth birthday, that was when he fell in love with me. Mind you, this was the man who said true love was a hooker that would take checks.

Ethel told us all, "It's Jack's birthday and we have to do something for him or we will all die a miserable slow death."

So I said, "What can I do?"

"Can you blow up these balloons?" she asked.

"'Till I am dizzy," I said and puffed out my cheeks to prove it.

I inflated the dozen or so black balloons which he always kept in his office. So then, after I blew them all up, the joke for months was "Anything that can blow that good has his heart." Well, there were a couple of balloons which stayed inflated for almost a year, so the joke continued to what seemed like forever.

Jack loved the way I adapted to the system. He respected the way I handled the clients and he learned to respect me. He filled in the gaps between my experience and my knowledge of addiction and the client's manipulation. He loved that I was such a quick study. In fact, at one point he actually bowed down to me stating that he had been humbled by my genius. He also said he had never before in his life seen anyone suck up, brownnose, or kiss ass better than him until he met me! Coming from the best con-artist I had ever met, this was a true compliment.

The first year and a half were just moments of debate between Jack and I. Some casual discussions, philosophical what-ifs, and a lot of BS. We had gotten comfortable with each other; the jokes, the clients, and the mutual dependency which forms in survival work situations. I was still pretty much a rule follower, then came *that* day. For weeks, Jack had taken up walking on his lunch hour and I agreed to walk with him. Lunch hour started at 10:00AM, so I worked until 10:00AM. He, on the other hand, had his walking shoes on at 9:50 and announced he was leaving, "Now." He was, at that moment, without a doubt the asshole he proclaimed to be. So, I thought if he was not going to wait for me, *to hell with him.* This was the message I got from him if I could not be on time.

Later that afternoon, we had a staff meeting and we had to get our monthly dispensing sheets out and into the charts. Being the team person that I am, I suggested we get to it. I was still full of rage over the walking incident. Jack had hurt my feelings and I was trying to find a way to hide my tears and my red eyes.

"They are out of alphabetical order," Jack shouted after checking the charts. "Who touched my stuff?" Now my dear friend went into a tirade.

I started to explain, "So, even out of order is a help, right?"

Mr. Asshole said loudly, "What am I supposed to do with these?"

I suggested he shove them, if his head was not in the way. We did not speak for months. It was hell on both of us, actually everyone. Talk about acting out, Jack made my client Chewy look like a gentleman! I do not remember why we started talking again, but what a relief for us all when we did. The kind of relief when you feel happy, safe, free, and complete.

As our conversations resumed, we took on a whole new level of trust. We even started to get personal. Once, he submitted that he loved me like a sister and that he knew I was living in hell. He began walking on eggshells around me, he was involved. The clinic staff knew of my separation from my husband and they witnessed my changing personality, so did my daughter.

Well, Jack knew, the staff suspected, it was like trying to hide a hickey from your mother! The truth was I realized I had been living in an abusive relationship with my husband. Some days I had bags under my eyes and other obvious signs. Hell, we *were* trained counselors, trained to look for these things. We saw the same signs and symptoms in our clients every day. Talk about denial! As it worked out, they all loved and enabled me. My husband had been out of the house for almost thirty days, what an awakening!

~ ~ ~

Many of the counselors asked if I had seen Karen lately, that she had developed an *attitude*. Since the abortion a few weeks ago, I had given her some space. She knew if she needed anything, I was always available. I spied Karen waiting in line. The staff at the clinic knew how I was with my clients and one of the dispensing nurses had passed Karen on her way back into the dispensing room and called me on the intercom, "Allie, are you busy?"

"No, not really, what do you need?" I asked her.

"Karen is in line for her dose and I think you should see her. Something is up and it looks bad," she whispered.

When you saw the same people every single day, you just knew when things were not right. This was the same dispensing nurse who had worked in methadone clinics for almost nine years, since she was eighteen years old right out of nursing school. She continued to say under breath, "If someone asks me what their dose is again, I just might lose it!"

I heard her announce to a client in line as I was walking away, "Jon, your dose is 80 fucking milligrams, the same 80 fucking milligrams you have taken every single day for the last nine fucking years. Now, don't ever ask me again!"

Many clients gave the nurses a bad time, others did not. For some it was, "Hey, I used that recipe for mole you gave me, it was great." But for the most part, it usually was, "Hey, you watered this down didn't you?"

We did put water in every dose which was initiated because the clients started licking the cups. It was easier to swallow and a little faster this way. Methadone comes in a very thick liquid form. We even received threats of their not getting the amount they were supposed to and they really could tell if we switched pharmaceutical brands, go figure. But cheat them… never.

So when Karen got up to the window, the nurse said, "There is a hold on your dose, I can call your counselor." On the intercom she announced, "Allie, Karen is here, do you want me to let her have her dose?"

I said, "No, send her up." Why take chances, right? I heard her run up the stairs, the door slammed and my window shook, it always did when the door slammed.

"Hey chill, what's with the door, you want the glass to fall out on me?" I said.

"What the fuck is the deal with holding my dose? I have to get out of here. You know my Mom will get pissed and I'll have to put up with her as well as you." Karen positioned her arms folded, ready for an argument.

I said, "Hello, this is Allie and what is your name?"

"Quit with the funny stuff, I am not in the mood."

"Sit down," I said.

"I don't want to and I don't have to," she stated as she folded her arms tighter across her chest.

"Okay, stand up." I turned around from my writing for the first time and looked straight at her, "Aren't we looking like something the cat dragged in? You look like hell. You're using and those are more than love bites on your neck. Does he use a rope or his hands?"

"That is none of your business," Karen said trying to hide her neck by tugging on her shirt collar.

"Sorry, but it is. I can see your neck from across the street and so can everyone else. You did not get dressed to come to the clinic for two weeks and you are losing weight. Look at you. And I am just supposed to ignore it all? Mike is coming around again, isn't he?" I asked flatly.

"What am I supposed to do? He gives me money and if I let him in, the rest of the family has peace. He is the father of my children," she argued again.

"So he is a sperm donor and a violent man. I guess you can't remember that childhood you told me about and here you are repeating the same life for your kids to mimic."

"I don't have to listen to this," she snorted.

"Yes you do, if you want your dose," I stated calmly.

"Okay, so I used," she admitted, "So what?"

"Do you want a dose increase?" I asked.

"What good will that do? I will still use," she flatly stated.

"You are right, sounds like a good pain management program to me. Do those hurt?" I asked pointing to her welts.

"No, not now. What do you want me to do?" Karen finally settled down.

I suggested, "What about using the restraining order that you have on him? What about going back to school or getting a job. What about just saying 'No' to drugs?"

"Yeah, right," she replied.

"Did you ever go back to the clinic for your checkup?" I asked her.

"No, I am okay."

"Yes, I can see that," I said as I looked her over.

"Can I go now?" she asked.

"Karen, I can't help you if you won't help yourself. I am here if you need anything."

"Can I go?" she got up out of her chair.

"Sure," I told her, "I will clear your dose." I stood up as she headed for the door and I headed toward the computer to release her dose.

"I am a dope fiend, what do you expect?" Karen shouted as she walked through the door.

"More!" I shouted back at her.

Karen continued her tumble to a new low. She apparently was picked-up for some crime but quickly released. Then Mike must have gone back to jail because a new man came into her life. This guy was real scum, not my words but everyone else's around the clinic. Karen's appearance showed that she was neither happy nor clean. Her mother asked her to leave the house and she lost her MediCal somehow. This usually meant the children were also removed from custody.

Karen soon was discharged from my caseload and was on the program as a private pay. I saw her but she no longer talked to anyone. She was in another world and she was *tweaked* most of the time. [Note: This is the term used when someone is always on the crack pipe, or some sort of methamphetamine use.]

She apparently had tried to get pregnant again because she had been in for testing every other day for a week I was told. Now she needed to get pregnant to get her MediCal reinstated, new child new start. Then one day there was such a big commotion, someone must have told detectives that Karen was on the program. We all believed it was her mother who leaked the information. I had no idea that the two men sitting at the foot of the stairs were undercover cops. As Karen was walking back to scumbag's car right after she obtained her dose, they got her. That was the last I saw of Karen. Her back was turned and she was cursing the clinic staff with her hands cuffed behind her.

15 | Helping "Ozzie Nelson"

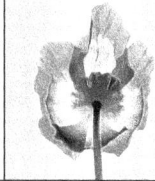

Dr. Green was one of those names that was in every chart. He was hated by the staff, he was a script-writer. Most of the clients at the clinic with MediCal saw Dr. Green. I thought he was a medical doctor (M.D.) until I saw one of his scripts for a client of mine, he was a psychiatrist. So I asked myself *Why does he prescribe cough syrup or Tylenol™ with codeine to methadone patients?* The other thing he did that I did not like was give the clients samples of antidepressants when there was no way for them to continue the prescription. Besides, no one ever thought about possible drug interactions. *So much for the medical establishment* I told myself.

Most of the clients liked Dr. Green, they went for counseling sessions with him when it was necessary. As Jack would say, "Right, like he can get them to talk more than we can?"

Many of my clients shared that they told Dr. Green about me, and I should go to work for him. I told them, "Thank you for the compliment but I am fine here."

Then the phone call came, "Is this Allie, the counselor I have heard so much about?"

I said, "That depends if it is good or bad news."

He said, "It is so good. I would like to meet with you for a business opportunity."

As if there was any privacy at the clinic—Javier was soon in my office asking why the doctor wanted to talk to me. He had evidently been in the office when the call came in.

I told him, "He said something about a business opportunity. When is my next review by the way Javier?" I think Javier thought I was joking but if there was a manager or director position, or the opportunity to create my own program, well, *adios* as they say in this neighborhood!

As it turned out, Dr. Green was opening a new clinic. He had his management in place, as well as, the program. He was very upfront with the fact that he knew if I came to work with him, several clients would follow. I told him for that type of position, I would remain loyal to my present employer. He did ask what my current wage and benefits package was, there was no way he could compete.

Later, I took advantage of our little meeting for my agenda too. I inquired about all the scripts he wrote and his response was, "What damage can a few T-3s do?"

I could never work for this man. We lost a few clients to the new clinic and mostly they were ones we wouldn't miss, although some of them eventually came back.

~ ~ ~

Eleanor was such a difficult case, she was now in very bad shape. Her liver illness was worsening and she was still in a wheelchair. With the guidelines many professionals must adhere to, it is difficult to actually decide what is physical or emotional abuse. This issue was just such a fine-line with Eleanor's daughters. At the time, as with many on my caseload, Social Services was involved as were the school districts. The oldest daughter was under the court's jurisdiction now, the daughters were abusing their mother. The stress level with adolescent children is bad enough but when you physically cannot help yourself, how can you help your children?

Eleanor was in-and-out of the hospital. It broke her heart to witness what her children were doing. Her eldest daughter had been given the opportunity to go to a juvenile camp but the youngest was now acting out. The relatives were helping themselves to her medications and, well, it was just a mess. We intervened in every way possible without breaking up the family because it was so very evident that Eleanor was not going to live much longer. Shortly after Eleanor's diagnosis, I thought she should have gone into an assisted living facility and the children into Foster Care. Some doctors are in a position to play God and it is hard for them to make wise choices for others. But she had managed to outlive all the doctors' expectations already by eighteen months.

~ ~ ~

It had been three days since I had received an email from Mom. I sent my brother an email and he confirmed what I thought, she was in the hospital. This was her first trip since the move. She had alluded to the fact that she was not feeling well and with her, a cold could go to dangerous places. She had gotten into a battle with the "daughter-in-law-from-hell" as she called her and that did not help either. I do not know what Mom expected when she moved, she had a new home and lots of land. She lived within the distance of a bike ride from my brother's house and we even joked about getting a motor for her wheelchair.

However, my brother's call confirmed my fears. I tried to speak with her but the nurse said he had just given her a sedative. He also said that she was difficult to handle and was not expected to live the night. Well, I had heard that one before. I made the phone call to my sister and called my brother who knew more than he had previously admitted. He stated he was scared and did not know what to do. As the big sister, I tried to reassure him that he was doing all the right things. Not one of us thought to call Mom's old doctor though. I did not sleep all night. As much as we had joked that one of these days she would die, it was different this time. Before when I arrived at the hospital in this area, early or late, I was allowed to visit her. I learned how to blend in so hospital hours or restricted areas meant nothing to me, but she was several states away this time.

I knew the auditor was going to be at the clinic for our surprise audit the next day. I had several charts to ascertain compliance which also meant Javier might show up early, or at least before noon. The coffee was on for hours when we had audits done. Everyone showed up and we were all grabbing our charts when I heard, "Allie, call on line four.

Who in the hell is calling me at this hour? I thought as I slammed the cabinet shut, then said out loud, "Oh shit, not now."

I guess it was the tone of my voice because for some reason Bonnie and Angie followed me. I picked-up the phone and just as I began, "Hey bro…"

He said, "She is gone Allie. I don't know what to do. Allie, she is really gone."

"Call your other sister," I said. "I will be on a plane as quick as I can. You did all the right things."

It was 4:40AM, a Tuesday and the auditor was coming. Everyone came in my office and said, "It's okay, leave now."

Jack and Todd offered me money. Ethel told me I had five days paid leave and not to worry *and* that the boss was here. Angie told me to give her my charts and everyone else told me to leave. I told them I needed to say something to Javier first. They were all so *there* for me.

I walked up to Javier and said in a very mean and cold voice, "My Mom did die this time. My charts are okay, Angie has them. My brother needs me and I am leaving."

He was stunned, I walked away. My displaced emotions were aired.

I closed my office and went downstairs to do something that I am sure was important. The clients were asking me for things but I was not me, not in my body. I thought *Pardon me, but my pain is more important than yours right now.*

I confirmed that I had five days paid leave. I must have appeared confused or looked scary because Moses grabbed me by my shoulders and said to me directly, "Whatever it is, it is, and it will be okay. Now go and take care of things and yourself. If you need anything call us and drive safe." It was then that I realized what a family we had become at our clinic.

Still in disbelief, I waited for the phone call which said, "No, your Mom is okay," but it never came. I confirmed with my brother that we were on our way and I would meet my sister at the airport, thank God for cell phones. I called my daughter and told her about her grandmother and that I was leaving. She was in the middle of senior projects so she could not go with me. I was uncomfortable with leaving her alone so I called my estranged husband just to let him know I would be away. Maybe I was looking for a shoulder to lean on, some sort of comfort, but I was hit with a request for reconciliation. Just what I needed at that moment, distraction.

I told him, "Give me a break, my Mother just died! How about just giving me some sympathy?" He retorted with how selfish I was. I managed to get to the airport by 10:00AM. I kept seeing the look on Moses' face and re-experiencing the strength of his hands on my shoulders when he said so seriously, "Whatever it is, it is, and it will be okay."

I lived ten minutes from an airport but due to my sister's fear of flying, I drove an hour in that morning traffic to meet with a frazzled woman on medication. She got panic attacks just thinking about flying, so out came the prescriptions. We both had on sunglasses covering our swollen eyes and were barely able to speak to each other. Thank goodness she brought her boyfriend who was not only able to get us on a booked flight, but managed to get us on the plane in twenty minutes. He later was able to get our Mom's estate settled in ninety days. It was the most horrible flight we had ever taken, no food and two layovers. Then we landed in the worst situation we could possibly have imagined, my brother's family.

My sister, brother, and I grew up children of a third-generation mortician family business. We certainly got some different perspectives on death because of it. However, my sis and I were not prepared for my brother's stepsons or the behavior of his wife and her family. I had not slept well the night before and I had been up since 3:30AM. The flight, I mean flights, were horrible and my sister was "out-of-it" the whole time. It was now about 11:30PM and I was exhausted.

The stepsons, seven and nine years old, wanted to throw Grandma's ashes in the Arkansas River with a bag of pennies. Of course, it had to be close to the Wal-Mart, her favorite place. We were used to joking about death, it was just never so close before. Since my Father's ashes had been placed in a sand-trap at his favorite golf course with a friend's ashes at his request, I wondered why the Arkansas River seemed so offensive to me!

My sister-in-law had been raised in the South and frequently used the N-word. Hey, but listen, it gets better! They took us to where Mom had lived, a brand-new house with brand-new things. The "sister-in-law-from-hell" asked us right that day if we would mind if her brother, who was getting married, could have what we did not want to take! I just told her we would talk about things in the morning. I was so glad that my sis was medicated, in fact, I almost wanted her to share!

The next morning, we were awakened by the sister-in-law and her mother and her sister who wanted to go through Mom's things. I thought this only happened in the movies! This was my brother's world, not ours. There was no "I am sorry for your loss" or "Can we fix you breakfast?" but instead "Can we pilfer the deceased's belongings?"

I looked at my bro and said, "Get us out of here before your other sister hurts someone." I had to pretend to be the stable one.

We had a marvelous day in Arkansas. We went to a mineral springs, soaked in the spa baths, and got massages. These were old clinics that were established during the civil war. It was a great place for three newly orphaned adults to rebond. I purchased a postcard of Bill & Hillary in front of a "Welcome to Arkansas" sign and mailed it to the clinic thanking them for their help. This also was my proof that I was really out-of-state just in case Javier had any doubts.

My sister and I spent the night going through Mom's belongings to decide what we wanted to take with us and what made sense to leave, which was almost everything. We could have stayed at least another day; but, secure in the thought that Mom would not end up in the Arkansas River, I thought it best to get my sister out of the state before she was arrested on murder charges.

We had an equally horrible flight home arriving at 1:00AM. I drove my sister to her house and returned to my own to find my estranged husband had decided to crash there, he was again cursing his sleep disturbance as I collapsed into bed. I was beginning to feel trapped in my estranged relationship. As I laid there, I could focus on some sort of escape to freedom, the freedom which I had experienced over the last month. Not the freedom like "Whoopee, I am single, I want to go out and party" but the freedom from the tension which is created by two people that have very different agendas.

At one point, I met with a dear friend, Dora, who just happens to be a therapist. She listened to me. She allowed me to explore my feelings, explode, and then regain some sense of normalcy. Anytime I wanted a little insight or to regain my sense of self, I went to lunch with Dora. She seemed to guide me forward, not backward, toward what was to unfold in my life. Dora is a true friend and spiritual sister. She knew I was getting burned-out with my job, however, I felt I needed that job more than ever now. I needed to escape my own life by focusing on others. Why is it so much easier to confront other people's problems? I figured, maybe if I ignored mine long enough, someone would come in and clean up the mess I had created in my life. So, back to the clinic.

~ ~ ~

Arturo was a rough looking character, the kind of person that would scare most of the straight society. He told me he was grateful to be out of prison. He had not intended to get back into using when he was released, but with five brothers that used heroin just waiting for him outside, how could he say no without causing family problems?

I intuited a sense of honesty, sincerity, and true remorse from Arturo. It was almost a useless effort on his part to even think, at this stage, he could live the straight life. But if that was his goal, I told him I would support his efforts. He had a long history of incarceration dating back to when he was twelve years old. This was the same age as most of my male clients' first incarceration. Evidently, his petty charges, when reviewed by the judge, added up to a lot of crime.

Arturo reviewed his story with me, also and his hopes and dreams. He really did not want much. As he stated, "I am thirty-five and it's time to grow up."

This sentence in itself was an admission of truth, which was so very rare. He was on probation, no driver's license, no job skills, and no education. He had his bike, his optimism, his woman, and their two-year-old daughter which he had just met. He wanted to become like Ozzie Nelson, the ruler of America's favorite sitcom family from 1952 to 1966.

I told Arturo I would help him in whatever way I could and started by giving him a copy of the want-ads from the local paper to support his job search efforts. I did not want to tell him right away that most of the employers which would consider him for employment would most likely do drug testing. Very few companies will hire employees on methadone. One could fight that decision but who has the resources? Different than most of the men at the clinic who had already surrendered to defeat, Arturo left the session feeling really good about himself.

Arturo even went out of his way to say "Hi" to me each day. He shared his job search efforts and let me see that he was not going to give up. Every day he rode his bicycle across three cities to get to the clinic and appeared to be committed to his goals. After being on the program for only four weeks, I received word from one of the counselors that Arturo was on the stairs and needed to see me. I opened the door and invited him in. He had been at the clinic earlier that morning.

"What's up?" I asked.

"I think I am in big trouble and I need your help," he said.

He had eluded previously that things at home were not in line with his fantasy of the Nelsons. Uncomfortable with the straight life and insecure with changes, he asked my opinion on things: "Is it okay for my old lady to steal in front of the children?" "Don't you think the baby should go to bed at the same time each night?" "I think I remember from a parenting class, but I didn't care then and I do now."

Arturo was struggling with his dream, his handicaps, and his efforts to be responsible. He had frustration with getting to the clinic early enough so he could provide his daughter breakfast and clean the house for the possibility of Social Services or the Probation Department to pop over. These agencies do not call and make appointments. He was also trying to find work on a bike. Another thing Arturo was concerned about was how his old lady and her seventeen-year-old daughter always had people over which he actually was afraid to have in the house. He knew they would just show up after he left.

I told him to have a seat in my office and went to get him a cold towel and a glass of water. It was a hot day and he was wilting. I came back, closed the door and said, "Okay, what's really up?"

"You said I could trust you, right?" he asked.

"Yes sir."

"You said if I needed anything, I could ask you, right?" he was sweating now.

"Yes sir, what happened?" I asked leaning over the desk.

He began to tell me that his old lady took the baby and her daughter and left last night about 9:00PM "She said they were going to a friend's house but she didn't get home until 9:30AM this morning," he almost cried. Then he related that they had "words" and she called the police on him.

I asked, "Did you hit her?"

"No, I swear to God and the life of my daughter. When she started throwing stuff and yelling, she hit me a couple of times. But like you said when that feeling come on me, I got on my bike and came here. She was on the phone when I left."

I was taken aback, I could only respond by nodding my head in support of his actions.

He continued, "If I go home, I go to jail. I can't do that. I ain't doing nothing wrong, but I know they won't believe me."

"What is she using?" I asked. His old lady was using the crack pipe he told me. I did not know what the correct action was but I said, "Do you trust me?"

He said, "Yes."

I reiterated the need for him to leave the area and asked if he had somewhere to go. He said he could go to his mother's house but then he could not come to this clinic anymore, also, there was the matter of his brothers. I told him there were other clinics and it was his choice. So I picked-up the phone and called the City Police Department. Oh, the look on his face!

I clarified to the lady on the other end of the phone that this was not an emergency but relating to an emergency call that they may or may not have just received. I explained I was a counselor at a Methadone Clinic and a client had just come from a situation who is on probation and is seeking guidance. The officer on the other end of the phone was shocked by my information and her tonality completely changed.

"Go on," she said, "yes, we did get a call regarding a domestic problem near the intersection you stated."

I said, "My client, rather than engage in familiar behavior came to me for help. Now, how can *we* help him?"

Her response was, "What does he want to do?"

I asked Arturo, "What do you want to do?" I had put the entire call on speakerphone to reinforce his trust.

"Can I get my things at home and leave?" he asked the officer.

The officer instructed me to have my client meet a patrol car at the intersection near the residence and he would be given a safety escort to obtain his things, there would be no legal consequence. Arturo told her it would take fifteen minutes to get home by bike and asked if they would wait for him.

She said, "No problem. Good job counselor."

I thanked the officer very much for her support and efforts, then hung-up the phone.

Again, the look on Arturo's face was complete shock. I told him, "You heard it and I am your witness."

He gave me a big hug and said, "Thank you."

I gave him a handful of business cards and added, "You might want these for the officers. Please call me and let me know what happens."

Well, Arturo called the next morning saying, "You should have seen her face when I walked in with the police and they gave her 'the business' and let me go! I am at my mother's house with the baby, they gave me a ride. I need to dose and can't get there."

I gave Arturo a few phone numbers to call for a clinic near him but they were all equally distant. I knew in my heart he would be using heroin again by morning, five brothers and all. So much for escaping *the life* and so much for his dream of the Nelson family.

I received two more phone calls over the next few months, one from Arturo's probation officer and the other from an attorney requesting a letter to help his client who was locked-up again. He was arrested for stealing milk and bread stating it was for his baby, it did not look good.

16 | Meditate versus Sedate

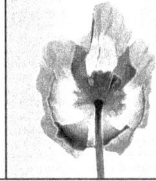

It was one of those mornings when I just wanted to stare out the window. It was cold and gray out, nothing really important needed to be done, everyone was sort of quiet. I stood watching the clients come and go, looking into their cars, checking to see who uses a seatbelt and who did not. This was the latest crackdown in the neighborhood, the tough seatbelt sting.

I saw Connie and her husband pull into the lot. He was a flaming jerk, real high profile and on Jack's caseload. Evidently, he threw a tantrum for everything and kept Connie under his control this way—an extremely abusive relationship. She was not even allowed to come up to counseling for more than five minutes at a time before the car honking could be heard from the parking lot.

I needed to talk to Connie but I did not have the energy to handle her husband's crap, besides she would not do what I told her anyway. She had MediCal because of the kids but he had to pay privately. It was fee detox time and he was most likely wigging-out. He also gave Angie a hard time about the letter for General Relief.

Why doesn't the jerk get a job? I wondered as I watched Connie get back in the car. Mr. Jerk got in after her. She picked-up a cup and, oh shit, she was spitting her dose out into the cup! Damn, she was giving him her dose. Well, that screwed up a perfectly quiet week. I went to the computer and put a hold on Connie's dose for tomorrow.

~ ~ ~

Troy was a self-proclaimed intellect. He did not get along with anyone at the clinic, staff or client. He just had a big blowout with Bonnie, his counselor. She once asked me if we could swap clients. It was not something that was done often but if it was obvious that a client needed to change counselors or be kicked-off the program, the counselor change was an option. I did not have anyone I wanted to trade, so I just offered to just take him.

Bonnie was always on the edge. She was severely depressed, with good reason. If there was a pile of crap, she would find it or it would land on her. Some people are just born victims, Bonnie seemed to be one of them. The day I met Bonnie, she showed me the scars of abuse from her childhood. Her husband had cheated and left her for the other woman. She now had their three sons to raise and a big mortgage to payoff. The boyfriend that she latched onto turned out to be a speed freak, always promising to cleanup and get a job. So, she really had four boys at home.

Javier drove Bonnie nuts, the clients drove her nuts, and she *was* nuts. She was always trying to diet but gained weight instead. The only joy in this woman's life was the dishwashing liquid under her kitchen sink! There was nothing that could separate her from her misery. So, if I could lighten her burden and get Troy off her caseload, it was my pleasure. Troy kept drinking alcohol and she could not get him to stop after three years of nagging. I took Troy's chart and put a hold on his dose for tomorrow.

~ ~ ~

Rebecca and Ruben were both on my caseload, they had been married for almost thirty-five years despite incarceration and the fact that Rebecca had developed a liking to women. They put on a good front and if you ran into them on the street you might have thought they were "the perfect couple" who just retired and were ready to buy a condo in Palm Springs. Ruben was wired tight, you could see the tension in his mouth when he talked. He was very short tempered and a know-it-all. He had a nasty past and was dangerous, my instinct told me. Rebecca always came up to talk, we got along fine but she did not get along with anyone else at the clinic. I think they thought they were better than the others.

Rebecca would discuss her childhood with me. She came from money, was a Jew for Jesus, and would not be in this mess if it was not for Ruben. She and Ruben would fight at least once a week. Their constant drug use and drinking did not help either. Ruben was constantly trying to get off methadone and so was she, but they never quit.

Rebecca was overly concerned with her looks. She walked for exercise, her hair and makeup was nice but the drugs and drinking had taken their toll. The worse addiction Rebecca had was her constant abuse of diuretics, she was always in-and-out of the hospital. I think it was the diuretic abuse that warranted most of it, or maybe the Valium, or the diet pills, or the drinking, or maybe the heroin. I allowed her to lower her dose because they were planning to move and she wanted off completely. Ruben had fee detoxed last week.

I do not know where my head was but somehow I missed the buildup of a feud going on at the clinic. Mary and her s/o, and Rebecca and Ruben, were at war with each other. Mary had been on and off my caseload over the last few months. She was on a run and her guy had been off the program for several months. He was such a sweet guy, once he noticed that my car window would not go up and came up to my office with some tools and offered to fix it. He needed the money and what the heck, it saved me a trip to the garage. He would not take the whole five dollars I offered, but took three stating he had borrowed enough from me over the years.

He asked if I had seen Mary.

Evidently, they had had one of their Friday night blowups and she wrecked the car. He had not seen her for a week and he was worried about her. The truth was he was lost without her, but much better off in my opinion. We talked about that fact but as usual, it was wasted breath. They were hooked-up again in no time, neither one on the program and that meant trouble.

When I first heard the word on what had happened, it was three days old. They said Mary and Rebecca had started it, of course, it was always the women. In fact, the only fights that ever happened at the clinic were with women, I guess it was the gossip and word-wars. Well, Rebecca got Ruben to go in and "defend his woman."

Ruben was arrested and I heard has a sentence of life in prison. Mary's guy went to the hospital for several weeks, serious injuries but lived. Rebecca was transferred to a clinic closer to the prison after the trial and no one has seen Mary. Thank God it happened on a Saturday when I was not here! It was the little things to be thankful for you know.

~ ~ ~

I first noticed Carla when she came to the clinic with an older man who drove a brand new Cadillac. Nice, new cars always caught the attention of the staff. It had to be either the auditor, DEA undercover, or a flashy client, and remember, we only had one of those. I had no interactions with Carla but we all knew who she was, we had a porno star on the program. It was rumored that she had brought a cassette of one of her movies but no one knew for sure.

Carla got on the program because she wanted out of the rut, however, I guess she got an offer she could not refuse. The director, producer, or the contract she negotiated included bringing her to the clinic daily for her dose. We were blown away because they brought her in a cab for her daily dosing and the fare was more than two hundred dollars! If she had been clean, she could have gotten take-homes. So, it did not take a genius to figure out that her heroin use would have been less expensive than the ride to the clinic—so much for our one celebrity.

Carla started on the twenty-one-day detoxification program and it was not working, she was assigned to me. She simply stated the man who drove her was a friend who offered to pay her bill. He looked about sixty to seventy years old, a widower most likely. Carla did not look bad for her age, not many tattoos or scars. She appeared to be very presentable when she had her teeth in. She was funny, intelligent, clean, and trying to put money away for her son's wedding. She was not on Welfare or Social Security, or "really working" as she put it.

During sessions, Carla asked questions about where to get this or that for the reception, or what did I think about this or that about the wedding.

One day, I had to ask, "So like you said, you do not work but this wedding has to cost a fortune. How will you pay for it?"

"Tricks," she said.

"Tricks?" I asked just to clarify.

"Yeah," she said but then defended herself, "I ain't working no street and I ain't one of those girls."

Carla told me she knew she did not have much longer to be able to "work" but needed to make as much money as she could now so she could buy her mom's restaurant. I joked with her that she must be good. She said that she had a few steady clients and this guy with the Cad was really good to her, he did not ask for much.

Then one day, Carla called me from the downstairs phone, "Look Allie, I got to talk to someone. I am gonna explode if I don't tell someone and you're the only one, can I come up? I need a favor too!"

"Sure, come on up," I said surprised. The wedding was over and she was clean, so there had not been much to talk about. Since I did not have a clue, I started to go through my referral files; prostitutes anonymous, shelters, etc. Also, we could handle any disease she might have. I thought I was ready for anything.

Carla came in with good energy and said, "You are not going to believe this shit. Never in my working life have I come across this. You remember that sweet old man in the Cad?"

I said, "Yeah."

"Well, he is a fucking pervert! Get this, I mean I been to his house lots of times. I know he has this other girl too, she is scum, I seen her out there. But get this, he wanted me to do it with his damn dogs! Can you believe this shit?" She shrieked.

My head reeled with thoughts like *I guess we all have our boundary lines, uh?*

I mean, what is a proper response to this? Not quite textbook stuff.

Carla broke my dazed silence, "I was so grossed out, I grabbed my money and walked to a phone booth and called a cab. I got the creeps, like I couldn't sit in his house and I sure didn't want to get in his car with him. Man, I gotta get a shower. Fucking pervert. I always wondered why he never wanted me to do anything with him, like he never fucked, wanted head, or anything. He paid me just to stay with him, gross. I wonder if that scum chick does it for him, gross to think of her with his damn dogs. I am gonna be sick. I gotta go. Here, I need you to keep this for me," she said and handed me five one hundred-dollar bills.

"I cannot keep this," I said.

"Sure you can. I just don't want to spend it and I will," she said as she pushed the bills back in my hand.

"What if I spend it?" I said with a laugh.

She said, "Use it and you'll pay me back, and if you can't, oh well. I just don't want to piss it away on dope and I will, if I have it."

"Okay, it is right here in my drawer. If I am ever not here and you need it, ask Jack." I told her.

"Okay, sure," she said walking out the door.

~ ~ ~

Connie's voice came on the speakerphone with attitude, "What is with the hold on my dose?"

I had forgotten about her, *glad I put the hold on it* I thought to myself. "Yeah, could you come up here for a minute?"

"I gotta go, my ole' man is here and he ain't in the mood," she barked back.

"Just get up here," I responded loudly.

"Can I dose first? It's a long line," she begged.

"I'll get you up to the window when I am done, okay?" A loud click was her answer.

Out of breath, Connie came blasting in, "What's up? I gotta go."

"You always gotta go, did your daughter make cheerleader?" I asked.

I wondered to myself *If she did, how would they pay for it? It cost me over a thousand dollars when my youngest made it on the team.*

"Yeah," she said, "that was two weeks ago."

I said, "Time flies when you're having fun, huh?"

"What do you want Allie, I gotta go?"

This was one of the times I could do what a normal methadone counselor was supposed to do, be an insensitive person; or, I could give her a chance.

"Are you aware of the consequences of dose diversion?" I asked.

"Dose what?" Connie said playing stupid.

"Dose diversion," I repeated and then defined. "When you do not swallow your dose, you spit it out, save it or give it to someone else, like a husband."

She went pale.

"You are damn lucky it was me that saw you and not someone else or I would have to do something. I was minding my own business up here looking out the window contemplating life, when I saw you spit out your dose and give it to Mr. Wonderful yesterday. So what's up? Tell him to get a job and pay his bill to get his own. Are you doing speed again? You have lost weight and your eyes are sunken in again!"

"Noooo, I'm not doing that again," she promises. However, her brother is on the program, one really bad dude. He was a big speed dealer. So it was not hard to figure out where she got it, especially being locked-up in the house all day.

I continued, "Quit acting like I am stupid or something, get off that shit. Again, tell your husband to get a job and pay his bill so he does not jeopardize your methadone. Unless you are ready to get off the program right now?"

Humbly she said, "I am sorry, I will."

"Will what?" I asked, "quit speed or tell your husband to get a job?"

"Both," she said.

"Okay, this is between us, okay?"

She said, "Thank you."

I reminded her that her actions were grounds for termination and just plain frigg'n gross. Connie laughed and I walked her downstairs.

Mr. Jerk was standing there and said, "C'mon, you have to leave, now. I have to go." Like it was something real important as usual.

We went to the dosing window, I watched her swallow and made her stand there for another minute talking so I knew he was not going to get her dose today. The bill was just paid so there should be no problem for a few weeks.

They were still fighting in the car when I returned to my office and looked out the window. He left rubber on the parking lot pavement, but I knew neither one would give me any trouble for a while.

~ ~ ~

"Troy here, you want to see me?" his voice beamed through the speakerphone.

"If you have the time, I would like to talk to you," I said.

"Sure, no problem."

"My office is next to the south exit," I explained.

"Okay," he responded.

Troy fell into the age group that is too old to be stupid and get into trouble and too young to not do anything. He was going to turn fifty in the next few months, so I thought we would talk about birthday presents.

I stood up and said, "Hello Troy, thank you for coming up to see me."

He told me he had seen me at the clinic for the last couple of years and had wanted to talk to me, so this meeting was great for him. He said he had been neighbors with Rebecca, they went to the same bar and she had told him about me.

"If it's good, it's true," I said, "and if it's bad, she is a liar."

He laughed.

I continued, "Bonnie came to my office yesterday, I guess you two had some sort of disagreement and she thought a counselor change might be in order."

"That bitch," Troy said. "For years I have tried to get a different counselor. I thought about switching clinics because of her but if my car breaks down I can take the bus to this one, so I never did anything about it."

"So you would be willing to accept me as your counselor?" I asked him.

"Sure," he replied.

"But I do have conditions," I warned.

"Okay, anything to get away from that woman. She is so depressing and she always watches me when I test."

I said, "Don't go there with me, okay? I won't bash my coworkers. She watches everyone just to make sure that someone doesn't cheat and get away with it. Do you have a problem with alcohol?"

"No," he said. "I happen to like it very much."

"You are a funny man. I am sure that Bonnie shared the information with you about Hepatitis C, right?"

"Of course, according to her I am a dead man waiting for the grave. So what difference does it make if I drink? I won't go to those damn AA meetings," he said.

"No problem," I said. "Why don't you take up religion, I understand that you read a lot."

Troy went on to tell me what a big player he had been, a dope dealer in the 1960s and 70s. Then he explained the big bust that made the news and how he knew everybody and had studied everything.

"So, do you meditate?" I asked.

"Sure," he bragged. "I studied with this guru and that guru."

"So why aren't you practicing your knowledge?" I asked him.

"That's a good question." he said. "I have been so busy fighting everyone's idea on what to do, I haven't been thinking straight. That is a good idea, I never even thought about it."

"A victim of your current circumstances no doubt," I said. "So you have studied EST?" [Note: This is a technique used in the 1970s coined by Werner Erhard; Erhard Seminar Training]

"Sure, I took that just before I went to jail," he affirmed.

"So, do you believe that your brain does not know if you are lying or not?" I continued this line of questions.

"Right on," he said.

"So, you are not an addict, or alcoholic, and can stop anytime?"

"Right on," he said slightly hesitant.

"Great," I say, "then we can plan your detox to be complete on your birthday and that will be a present to yourself, right?"

Beads of sweat formed on his forehead as he leaned over and said, "Let's see, my dose is now 50 milligrams. My birthday is in five months, that's 10 milligrams down a month. Kinda fast but I want to try!"

"Try? What is try? It is or it is not, you took the course. Are you making a commitment or not to being free of methadone by your birthday?" I asked him, pushing the issue harder.

"Doc won't let you lower my dose, Bonnie said so," Troy offered with a hint of defense. "I have asked her for a long time."

"Give me a clean test next week and there will be no problem," I instructed. "I will use your liver disease diagnosis as the reason. If you are clean, I can work with you."

He seriously looked at me and said, "I'll quit drinking, dope, and methadone, but I ain't gonna give up my pot!"

"Your choice," I said.

"But what about the tests?" he asked.

I said, "What about them?"

"Won't it show that I'm still dirty with pot?" he asked with concern.

"Can you keep a secret?" I asked leaning forward.

"Sure," he said like he was hearing the mystery of life.

"We don't test for marijuana," I whispered.

"You're kidding me?" he asked in disbelief.

"Nope, too expensive," I replied. "So, I hear that you have committed to getting off the program for the big 5 0 and that you are not going to consume liquor any longer, is this correct?"

Troy nodded and we shook hands on it.

"God, I feel great, this was great! I can't wait to get home and pull out my old books. I haven't read that EST stuff in years," Troy exclaimed with excitement in his voice.

"There is a reason for everything," I said sarcastically, "when the student is ready, the teacher appears." I made a face with my mouth wide open and my index finger in it like I was gagging myself, then added, "By the way, do you have a computer?"

"Yeah," he said, "I'm online too."

"Why don't you start researching treatments for Hepatitis?" I suggested.

"Wow, what an idea, I'll get on that right away. I never thought about doing that, thanks Allie."

"Now, don't get busted for pot either, okay?" I teased.

Troy laughed all the way down the stairs. The man was now empowered and I had to admit, I felt good about it too. Not often did I get the chance to open the door to a breakthrough, but we did it together that day.

It was hard-going with Troy sometimes, he was so full of himself and cocky. But every month we kept lowering his dose. He wanted to speed it up but I said, "Why rush things and create a possibility of a problem?" I acknowledged him for coming down as fast as he was and considering his health, why take risks?

The big test came when Troy's father died. The family had rejected him long ago due to the drug related problems. Back then his personality was not the greatest. As he put it, "An ego with an asshole, or an asshole with an ego." We talked about self-worth and self-pride after his father died. Troy assured me that he knew what he was doing and if his family wanted to hold on to the past, that was their choice.

The EST seminar work which Troy and I had shared, created a more structured language between us. We had no gray areas, everything was black or white. This was a powerful tool and anyone who has done the work knows what I am talking about. If Troy had an upset, I would ask him, "Why do you give that significance?" If he started negative talk, I would ask, "How does that serve you?" This type of dialog put everything back on him, it was his choice, his responsibility.

Troy got past most of his physical symptoms with the use of pot. We discussed the commonality of switching addictions and how he could not afford to be stoned all the time—either spiritually, physically, emotionally, or financially. I suggested he meditate versus sedate.

Just before Troy got off the program, he even took a vacation, the first one in years. It was the best time he could remember, this motivated him even more. Due to the difficulty in getting take-homes with all the hoops he had to jump, he wanted his freedom from the program real bad.

His last dose was the day before his birthday, he cried when he thanked me for helping him find the way to his freedom. He even went to find Bonnie to tell her it was his last day, he thanked her for her efforts over the years. She later came to my office with tears in her eyes, she could not believe that Troy thought enough of her to thank her and say good-bye. Bonnie asked me what I did for him that she could not do.

"I just served him his own BS," I told her. I tried to explain the EST seminars to her but she did not get it.

I do not know for sure if Troy is still clean or sober, but I get a Christmas card every year that says, "Thank you again for my freedom, doing good, Troy."

17 | Dope Never Lies

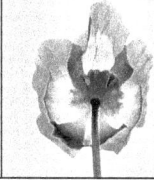

Eleanor was not doing well at all; she was missing doctor appointments, not clearing her medications, and had not gone to get a test performed. I was short with her because there was no reason for transportation to be a problem. For two years, I gave her forms which I could not fill out, but if she did she would get free rides. Then she asked me if I would make out a will for her and if she had made the right choices concerning her girls and money. Not that she had any money, but she did have small savings accounts for her girls.

I asked Eleanor about her oldest daughter and she stated at this point it was a lost battle, she had lost control over her. It actually surprised me that she knew she had to make the call to the probation officer to report this and did. The report kept her out of trouble for only thirty days, she had a boyfriend. Eleanor thought he would be good for her, keeping her off the streets and all. She said that he lived upstairs, was nineteen, and seemed like a "good boy." Personally, I did not think there were any "good boys" around for at least ten miles in any direction.

Values, what is right? What is wrong? Eleanor tried to send her daughter to the grandfather's home in Mexico, that did not work. She tried to have her stay with her father and his wife, that did not work. She sent her to a cousin's house in the Valley to do childcare, that did not work. The girl had also gone to a Juvenile Detention Camp, that just made things worse.

Eleanor explained that her daughter could not go to school because the continuation school did not start until the ninth grade and she was still considered a sixth grader! Homeschool was not working, no one could make her study. So, Eleanor told me about this great boyfriend that was in between jail time (assumption on my part) and who she thought would control her daughter.

I just said, "Who knows…" I did tell Eleanor that if she did not get to the doctor soon, I was going to go medieval.

I took some flack when I removed her take-homes in a power play, it was a tough call on my part, but it worked. Some of the other clients had things to say about my decision when they heard, but they knew me well enough to understand that I had a reason. Many of the women had gone over to Eleanor's home to try to help, but there was not much anyone could do.

I told these women, "If you are so concerned, you take her to the doctor, get her tests done, get her prescriptions, and help straighten out that daughter." Well, that was the end of any further complaints from the so called "concerned" clients.

I removed Eleanor's take-homes and made her come to the clinic every day. Sure it was hard on her but she needed to get a medical test done, as well as, get her prescriptions refilled. It took her two weeks and I knew it did not take that long to get the appointment. Afterward, her take-homes were reinstated immediately. So, was I that horrible or had I manipulated a few more months of life for her?

~ ~ ~

I just really wondered what's really going on? This was the question Moses would ask me at least once a week, if not daily. I looked at the number of drug programs and listened to the stories of abuse within the systems. From the police to the jails; from the halfway houses to Foster Care; and, even in treatment programs, there were overworked case managers in every field of human services. I saw the benefits and I saw the traps.

I asked myself many times, *how am I supposed to rehabilitate a person who wants to be rehabilitated? And does he or she really want to be rehabilitated or is he/she there just because they have to be? Do we really understand the depth of rehabilitation?* It was not just that they needed to be trained to do a specific task like coming in for dosing, it was that they could not get up and out on time everyday to do it. This type of responsibility and training starts when one leaves the womb. So, does it begin with the parents?

How do you support change without compromising individuality? How do you teach the thirty-year-old woman with a fifteen-year-old daughter that school was more important than boys when she never finished school and had her daughter at the same age? The teen feels she is doing all right, just like her mother did, right?

How do you teach a boy to be a man and that machismo has nothing to do with it? And how do you tell him to keep his pants zipped so he does not become trapped like his father? How do you motivate this young man to stay in school and get a job when he can make so much more money selling dope on the street? Besides, the schools do not want these kids there anyway. How crazy have things gotten that children are kicked-out of school for things that used to be controlled by detention? When did we lose control?

How do you stimulate people to look at their family of origin, the behaviors and the consequences, and still keep their self-esteem while not totally alienating them from their roots? How do you teach people to dream, to set goals, and encourage the discipline to achieve them at the age of twenty, thirty, forty, or sixty when they may not actually stand a chance? How do you get them to give up an excuse of addiction which society continued to use against them and that has a better payout than sobriety? Pain sucks and there is a lot of it in *the life*. How do you teach people to tolerate the pain?

Once sobriety is achieved there is guilt, remorse, and shame to deal with like the new behaviors, new speech patterns, new thought processes, and even job training to master. These clients still had children at home, rent to pay, possibly a spouse with which to deal, and we expected to change them? Do we legalize everything or just keep putting everyone in jail and their children in Foster Care?

Just think about the number of people out there who are using and the number of children who are abandoned emotionally and physically; now, think about those numbers abandoned not just by heroin addicts but by working parents? The kids are angry and who can blame them? Anger is contagious and this is how the pain free escape called "addiction" is created.

"Just Say No" the slogan goes. "Ha!" these people laugh in our faces.

We, the mothers and fathers who pay the taxes for most of the services in place, we, the ones popping Prozac, Viagra, diet pills, sniffing sinus medication with our light beer or White Zinfandel while still smoking our cigarettes, we are the ones who are not there physically or emotionally for society's kids.

Of course, the family unit is there for them. There are plenty of stepmothers and stepfathers; boyfriends and girlfriends; new grandpas and grandmas; and, of course, there is always Ritalin. Maybe the little buggers really cannot sit still in class because there is no structure at home, but guess what, dope and alcohol is there for them and it never lies, it never breaks a promise.

Bev and her husband had been on the program for many years with sporadic periods of abstinence. They had two teenage children. Bev came to me with problems at home and I asked her about the kids and school. Her son, fourteen, had already been expelled from junior high. She could not make him get to his continuation classes, which were all of three hours a day.

My first thought was *What the hell is wrong with the school system that they could not keep a problem kid in school for seven hours? What happens the rest of his day if he attends school only three hours?* So, our schools put the ones out on the street which they could not control, and obviously, the parents could not control them or they would not have been kicked-out of school in the first place. How can we help make parents more responsible? Well, maybe we make them sit in class all day to take care of their kid!

"Why can't he get up to go to school?" I asked Bev.

"He stays up all night with his girlfriend," she replied.

"Is he having sex?" I asked afraid of the answer.

"Oh, sure," she said. "My husband and I have argued about this all the time. It's safer for them to be at our house than on the street."

"So, your husband has encouraged your son to bring his girlfriends over for sex?"

"Yes, I guess so," Bev answered lowering her head.

"How old are the girls?" I asked.

"Oh, I guess they are his age, thirteen or fourteen, they are nice girls," Bev replied.

"Do their mothers know their girls are having sex?" I continued the questioning.

"I don't think they care, they never said anything," Bev explained.

"What about your daughter, is she having sex too?" I asked.

"I don't think so, but maybe."

"Aren't you concerned about this?" I kept quizzing her.

"How can you stop it?" she said. "They just get to an age and you know you can't tell them anything."

"What about drug use?" I asked.

"Oh, my son I know smokes pot. My husband doesn't care. 'At least he's not using speed,' he says to me."

"Is that okay with you?"

"No, but what can I do about it?" Bev asked with more concern in her voice.

"What do you think?" I asked already knowing this line of questioning was getting nowhere fast.

What can I do? I thought to myself. Here we have a family with the Probation Department watching the father; the Department of Children's Services monitoring the children and the mother; the school district involved (supposedly monitoring attendance); and, the Juvenile Justice System spying in because I later discovered the boy had already been in trouble with the law. What *can* I do?

~ ~ ~

Cindy lived across the street from the clinic, she had been on the program for several years. She was hard to miss, if she had her hat on she looked like a fifteen-year-old boy. I saw her frequently with her son who was adorable. We got to watch many of the children grow-up, Cindy's son was a clinic baby. I watched Billy grow from a baby being carried to the clinic, his first steps trying to walk up the stairs, to riding his hot-wheels to get his daily "special water" while mom received her dose. Cindy came to the women's group when we had them, she always brought Billy with her who was very well behaved.

When Cindy was transferred to my caseload, I was shocked when I reviewed her chart. She was actually thirty-five years old and did not look a day more than twenty, without her hat on. She had a total of six children, Billy was the only one she had custody of, she would not risk losing him. Cindy was clean as long as she got to the clinic on time and she stayed away from her family, this was difficult since she still lived at home.

My goal, believe it or not, was to get Cindy to the clinic each day to get her dose. Living across the street, she usually arrived at 12:28PM having just woken-up. I suggested that there was no excuse to be late, she said she needed her sleep. I suggested that she go to bed early; she asked who would watch her son if she went to bed early? I said the boy should go to bed early too, she said she did not think of that. So we tried to make her dose time before 10:00AM with the goal of no more no shows, then she would get a take-home.

Sadly, Cindy was a victim of family incest, not an uncommon history within this population. It had been her uncle. Her parents were born to immigrants with a strong work ethic and foreign cultural values. They had worked twelve to fifteen-hour days and left their children at home with the grandmother who did not speak English, this was such a common thread. No one ever questioned the children's school attendance, or their timeliness. If there was ever a need for her father to go to the school, there was a beating, you did not embarrass the family. After a few beatings, you were kicked-out of the house and then hung out with friends and watched television all day. As long as the chores were done, nobody said much. After all, like Bev said, "What can you do?"

Cindy had gone through a great counseling program and understood how she got where she was, she did not blame anyone. I was trying to find a spark to motivate her to just get up and get dressed in the mornings. I asked her about having her own home.

"Why?" she asked.

"You can work," I said. "Is there any work you would want to do?"

"Why?" she asked.

"Don't you want to go to school?" I asked trying not to get discouraged myself.

"Why?" she asked. She said she had a home, she had food, she could stay with her son, and she did not need money. "So what is your point?" she asked.

"Well," I said, "my job is to motivate you to get off drugs and keep off drugs. So if you don't do something, you will do drugs, right?"

"Not necessarily," she said.

"Isn't methadone a drug?" I asked her.

"Yes," she admitted.

"I want you to quit taking methadone too," I told her.

"I don't think so," she said, "that just won't happen. It's the only way I can keep from getting strung out again."

Cindy had artistic talent, so I suggested that she market her drawings. I had printed information on Latin Art and biographies of lesbian artists to stimulate her imagination. She showed a glimmer of interest when I discussed the Mayan culture and how it predicted women were to come into power in 2012 or so. I explained how her art could be a way for her to come into her *own* power. She politely accepted the material but nothing came from it.

I really had a hard time demonstrating restraint the day Cindy came to my office to vent. "What the hell is wrong with these kids today?" she asked. "I mean, why aren't they in school? Why don't they get it? It's all fucked up out there."

"What happened Cindy?" I asked with concern.

"Well, first of all it's my sister. She is tweaking all the time and I am afraid for my nieces. She is always losing her temper and I hate the way she yells at them. She has no patience with the baby, I think it was born on crack. But if that's so, then she wouldn't have had her, right?"

"Most of the time," I said avoiding the topic.

"Well, the kids got in her purse and her shit spilled all over the place. I saw it and got it cleaned up before our mom saw and before the girls got into it, thank God. Then I beat the shit out of her for being so stupid and now mom is pissed at me! So then I walk to the market, right, and I run into my oldest daughter who lives by there. I haven't heard from her in months and she goes and asks me for money to buy a dime bag. I send her money all the time, now I find out she is into this shit! You'd think they would have learned from me. Like, that's why I let them go, so they wouldn't turn out like me! Things are all fucked up," she ended almost in tears.

All I could say was, "That's why you need to get out there, Cindy. Start a group, go around and talk, teach the children *your* lessons."

"I tried Allie, I even went to Eleanor's house to help with her girl. Man, that chick fell fast into the life, she don't listen to nothing."

"Call Child Protection on your sister," I suggested.

"That's heavy," she said, "but I think I will. I can't believe she is so stupid, that bitch. But... then I'd get stuck watching her brats."

"Get a job and you won't have to. Get a place of your own and you would not have to worry. Do something besides watch television, Cindy," I said trying not to sound condescending.

The next week she came with a job application for a janitor position in the school district. I helped her fill it out. A few days later, she told me she turned it in and that was the last I heard about job search efforts from Cindy for a while. Then shock of shocks, one day she casually announced she took a night job at a food packing plant so she could be with her son during the day. The job lasted for three weeks. The management did drug testing on all their employees and she was found to have methadone in her system. Cindy was let go due to company policy.

18 Learning to Expect More

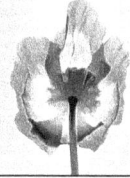

"Allie," the voice came over the speakerphone.

"Yeah," I responded.

"The doctor wants you to come down and help with a medical patient, she doesn't speak English and it appears to be a domestic violence problem."

"Sure, right there," I said.

So, in my very best Spanglish (half-Spanish and half-English) I tried to get information from a woman whose face had been used as a punching bag. She was afraid that she was going to be punished because she was an illegal alien. She was told by her neighbor that this was a safe place and we would not report her.

Once we got past her fear of immediate deportation—which could have been a blessing for this poor woman at this point—we tried to direct her to a safe place with instructions to call the police if her husband did this again, all the while knowing she would go home. She did not work, did not speak much English, had no money, did not drive or have transportation, and had two infants which were with a neighbor for safety. Domestic abuse was one of the toughest things to deal with and seem all too frequently with drug and alcohol abuse. We attended this woman's medical needs, gave her all the referrals we could, and then let her limp away.

~ ~ ~

Dolly had just moved to California, so she was transferred to our clinic. She and her husband had been married for twenty years and using heroin for almost forty. When I looked at her, I understood what they meant about the effects of heroin. Heroin, when used safely does not harm the body the way many drugs do. But it is the lifestyle and desperation which caused the problems. Dolly actually looked pretty good for her age but you could see pain in her eyes. She said the first time she used heroin was right after her mother died, she had no idea her brother was also into it.

At the time, Dolly was in such emotional pain that her brother's girlfriend told her she had something that would take the pain away, it worked she said. This was something Jack kept telling me, the problem with drugs was that they worked. Dolly learned that her brother's girlfriend just wanted another female to get high with, she said the rest was old history.

"Look," she said, "don't think you are gonna change me, I am too old to change. I don't use no more either, so don't worry about that. I just take my 40 milligrams and get on with my day, okay?"

I said, "You just might become my favorite client."

She asked, "You never got into this shit did ya?"

"Nope," I said.

"I can tell, you're different. You know me and my ole' man, we been around here a long time, we know just about everyone. We used to be the testers for the new shipments, you know, to tell the quality of the stuff? Ain't been no good stuff in a long time, not like we used to get. I even helped get a Methadone Clinic approved a few years ago. I went around to all the stores trying to tell them people on methadone not to steal no more, it would be a good thing and all to get a clinic close by."

"So, Dolly, when was the last time you went to the doctor?" I asked.

"Well, I see Dr. Green but that is for something else. I need to go but I am afraid, I think I found a lump in my breast. I don't think I can handle the answer," she said touching her chest.

I started to share my own story stating I knew just how she felt, I was there several years ago. I broke the tension by telling her that the lump I had was how I found out I was pregnant.

She said, "God no, I took care that. I didn't bring no kids into this life knowing I used heroin. These women who keep getting knocked-up piss me off."

"Good for you," I said.

"Go ahead now, tell me your story," she said, "I don't have to go yet."

So, I told her, "My Grandma had her breast removed due to cancer but the cancer returned and she died. So when I was twenty-four and found a lump, I went straight to the doctor. He said to come back after my next period but I didn't have one for nine months because I had a baby instead! Well, the lump disappeared.

Afterward, with all the talk about getting mammograms, my husband got on my back. I didn't want to go, I agonized for two years. Then I told myself 'what the hell' because I could feel the lump again. So, for my fortieth birthday, I did it. I figured whatever was to be, would be. The radiologist said he was not supposed to but he read my x-ray before I left and said it was nothing. I cried all the way home. So, Dolly, go do the test."

Then I had Dolly do a mind game. I told her to keep telling herself it was nothing, and it would be. Her mind won, she went for her test and it was nothing and I had a new friend.

The next thing Dolly and I worked on was to get her to stop smoking. She had a bad cough but refused to give up her cigarettes. She was a sweet sweet woman, the adoptable kind. I got her to lower her dose by 20 milligrams, that was about the best she would do. She had been "to hell and back several times" she reiterated but with no details. She was just "a sweet lonely lady now."

I tried to find things for Dolly to do just to get her out of the house, she found a way on her own. At least once a week, she and her husband got on the bus and took a day trip to nearby casinos so she could play Bingo. It was what she lived for, thank goodness for Bingo!

~ ~ ~

Joey was the youngest person on the program, that I knew of. I also had his father and did have his uncle on my caseload, at one time. Joey had gotten in a car accident and it destroyed his arm, he was in a lot of pain and his uncle found a solution for him. We had no intention other than to ease the pain, but the pain medication became too accessible.

Due to missed school, no mom in the home, and a dad that worked all day, Joey took to the streets. He later was shot in the same useless arm, it still hurt so the pain medicating began again. This time he scored his own medication, heroin- Joey himself chose to go on the program, after all, his dad and uncle were on it. They could not give up the habit, right?

It took a while but Joey became a clinic project. A few of us gave him the business whenever we saw him: "Hey, get a job" or "Hey, get in school" or "Hey, get away from those girls" and "Nice haircut, now if we could just get you in long pants." The poor kid had more and more people telling him what to do. He did receive plenty of benefits but he was under the impression that he was "handicapped" and could not do anything but collect Social Security.

Joey was actually on Todd's caseload, there was a reason for everything. Todd became the surrogate parent that Joey had always wanted. Not to put down his father but he only knew what he knew. The man held a job, a good one, and he did not bring women home. His wife had died when Joey was a baby (no details) and he raised the boy the best he could. He had no idea that his brother was slipping the kid heroin for pain management but the pain was not as bad as the medicine was good. Joey's uncle had no intention of ruining the kid's life, but maybe the mistake in his efforts cost him his own.

In a session one day with Joey's uncle, I said, "Do something different today, okay?"

He said, "Look, I am a fucked up addict, I even got my nephew hooked on this stuff, that's how fucked up I am. So like, just don't expect me to be anything more than a dope fiend and we will get along fine."

This statement told me a lot. I never discussed it with Joey's dad but the uncle and I decided we were going to encourage Joey to get back into school. He did just that! It took a couple of tries before it stuck but the two of us did not cut him much slack. We both asked for report cards, test scores, and offered to help him study. We even taught him how to buy a computer and use it. Joey just needed the attention and we both needed someone to succeed at something.

It was so hard to teach someone how to be different, to shed the self that is known and familiar and dare to be something more. It is hard for them to feel the fear and do it anyway. It is difficult to look at what you have, and think about what you want. Joey went through all these emotions.

How do you make someone hungry for something that they have never tasted? To help them develop a taste for that bittersweet success that the straight life has to offer? Do we do it by encouraging self-pride and comparing situations of the absurd with which they can relate when the payoff is not always as good, even if it is temporary?

At this point, fears and questions rise up within them, "If I get a job, then I have to go to work every day and I might get fired, then I lose my benefits!"

"Then you get another job," I would respond.

"But I could get fired again and they expect me to do all this for minimum wage?" they would ask me.

Then they would say, "Figure it out Allie, I don't get no MediCal benefits for ninety days and what if I get sick? How do I pay my methadone bill? What about drug testing? Who will watch the kids? I can't trust them daycare centers, ya know? And what if the baby gets sick and I miss work and get fired? No, it's better I just stay home."

"Then go to school, take one class at a time," I would suggest.

They would come back with, "Yeah, but what for? No one is going to hire me, I did time. I done that Gain Program, they gave me clothes and stuff and they even had childcare, but it was too much for me. To get all the kids in school, the baby to daycare, me to the methadone clinic, then to a job? Who are you kidding? I would worry about where the kids went after school, need to pick up the baby and all on the bus? What, and you want me to fit in exercise too? Yeah, right. Sorry Allie, maybe when the baby is in school and I get a driver's license and a car. I think I should just find me a better man to help me pay my bills." Ah, the path of least resistance.

Another point to consider when trying to help someone is the fact that he or she will most likely have a legal history which may trigger drug use. And it may instigate making another baby which brings more domestic confusion for the kids. Then he or she will get arrested again and life goes on, and on. Trying to rehabilitate society forty to fifty people at a time as on a common caseload was tiresome. Especially, when society will not forgive, forget, or get with a game plan. One day at a time I told them, one goal at a time. Forget about your loneliness, forget about your family and friends, forget what is comfortable, just try a *different direction*.

We need an Addict Relocation Program, like the federal Witness Protection Program with an instant new identity, an instant new life. There *is* a program somewhat like this. They take up to two children under the age of four and their mother if she is below 40 milligrams, but getting to the 40 milligrams is the hard part.

Then the questions arise again: "What about the older kids?" "What about the few belongings that I do have?" "Who will take care of my mother?" "What about when their father is released?" This was a lot to ask of a person. Would you be willing and able to just uproot your entire life if asked?

~ ~ ~

Donnie just turned twenty-two, he had been in some sort of system since he could remember. He was put in Foster Care as a baby, not remembering or knowing his mother or father. He thought he was a crack or alcohol baby, that was what they told him anyway. Donnie remarked once, "I think I took to drugs because I took that stuff when I was a kid, you know, Ritalin?"

He had never been with one family very long. He had been to several schools and juvenile halls up and down the coast. Donnie finished up his time at the California Youth Authority just eight months ago. This was the longest he had been out of any system that he could remember.

Donnie "lucked into a job" at the carwash and had a new woman. She got pregnant right away, now six months along. He said he did not mind that she had three other children, it was the family he always wanted.

"Yeah, she is gonna get on the program too," he stated, "as soon as we get her to a doctor for the baby."

"Great," I said.

"The only problem is, she is mean. She gets mad at me all the time, she is real good with the kids but, man, she got a temper. I guess it's because of being pregnant and all. I just want to do the right thing for her," Donnie explained with compassion.

This sounded like reverse domestic abuse to me. Covered in his love bites with one child on his arm, we talked about what needed to be done for the kids. We talked about how he could help with the chores, and what was acceptable and not acceptable in the way of fighting around the kids. I instructed him that when it started to get ugly, go for a walk or let her go for a walk. Also, to offer to watch the kids for her sometimes. Take turns coming to the clinic and give yourselves short breaks from the children.

The first downfall for this couple was when their car got towed for expired tags. It was just as well, neither Donnie nor his woman had a driver's license or insurance. But now they had to buy bus passes or walk to the clinic. Looking back on it, I think maybe it was the wrong thing to suggest coming separately to the clinic. The woman had a jealous streak and she thought Donnie was getting too friendly with another woman at the clinic.

Angie reported that her client had been threatened with a knife and there were tires slashed. So, Donnie's woman needed to transfer to another program. The transfer never happened, she was arrested and the children were placed in Foster Care. Donnie was fee detoxed from the program and that was the end of that. Hopefully, his life decisions changed in a more positive direction over the next few years.

~ ~ ~

"Halleluiah and praise the Lord Jesus Christ! AAAmen Brother, Jesus will forgive your sins. AAAmen Brother, Jesus will heal you!! AAAmen Brother, Jesus will love you! AAAmen and praise God. Brothers and Sisters hear us, join us, love is the answer! Praise the Lord Jesus Christ!"

There was one man preaching and then came a group, "AAAmen!"

It was Friday morning about 5:20AM, still dark with the normal line at the front door. The parking lot was full and I did not recognize who was doing all the yelling on the corner. Four or five of them were praising Jesus as loudly as they could.

"Hey Jack, what's up?" I asked.

"Don't know yet Allie, just going to punch my time card and mosey on out there. It's like they know when Moses isn't around. Come on out with me and lets bask in the Glory of God this fine morning," he chuckled.

Jack and I crossed the lot to introduce ourselves.

"Hello Brother, Hello Sister, and how are you this beautiful day? Praise God, Amen," the man said.

"Wishing it was a little quieter," Jack said.

I said, "Hey look, we don't mean to stop your good work here but this is a residential area and as important as your task is, I don't think these people would celebrate your inspiration this early in the morning."

"I don't think we want the police here either," Jack chimed in.

We suggested they go ahead and come inside for a half hour of recruiting and then go on their way.

"But, I have the spirit of the Lord and I need to share with all God's children the gift of forgiveness and healing that the Lord our Savior Jesus Christ has to offer, Amen!"

The rest of the group shouted, "Amen Brother!"

"I want to share in your Evangelism but you must, and I do insist, that you most immediately do it much more quiet." I tried to keep it friendly, the last thing we needed were picket signs around the clinic!

It was bad enough what went on here, but to reject God, well, we did not need that added to our agenda. They came in for a while but were so disruptive we had to ask them to leave peacefully. We suggested they leave outreach information and we agreed to put it in the lobby right next to the Planned Parenthood flyers and HIV services information. They were not real happy but left peacefully.

We just hoped the neighbors did not react, we were always on edge with them. A couple of residents complained about the parking in front of their houses which I mistakenly did when I first came here. After all, you could not park in the parking lot, remember? One poor man had his house on the market for over a year before it sold. Would it have made a difference if it was just another type of medical clinic that served the poor? Probably. No one can be blamed, but where do you put a program like this?

We were really pretty lucky, some of the clinics were not located in good areas at all. The clinics need to be accessible and the clients need to learn to acclimate. Clients want treatment, they actually want to meet the challenge, if the challenge is available. When we added time for increase counseling, it was worse than pulling teeth to get them to the clinic and sit for fifteen minutes twice a month. But when these clients had to sit for an hour a week things really changed. Others made sure they got their session and it was not just to talk about the latest television show, even though many times, that was a good start. Important issues were talked about once the clients felt heard.

Many clients expressed the same indignation as the inmates that I had worked with, they asked, "Why should I talk to you? Like, you can change something? What do you get out of this?"

Once they felt safe with you, they began to trust and allow me to hear their stories which are so very personal. We heard stories of real life, real feelings, their humiliation, and their pain. So much of what needed to come out was buried so deep and was way too painful to relive ever, far less now. Many professionals have a vision of a client in session nodding-off or drooling as they come onto their dose. Sure, people on methadone can be demeaning in their tonality, but try to counsel in between nods? No, it was not like that. I was once told that after working in a methadone clinic, my professional career would be shot. I guess they thought heroin was just going to go away or all the drug users would one day be abducted by UFOs.

19 | Too Close to Home

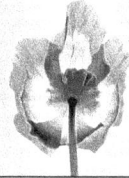

"Allie, call on line three," Ethel's voice stated on the loudspeaker.

"Thanks, Ethel," I said as I pushed 3. "Hello, this is Allie."

"Allie?" a soft voice asked.

"Jackie? Hi, what's up? You are crying," I knew my close friend's voice.

"Guess who I just caught smoking pot?" Jackie asked me.

"One of my girls?" I asked.

"No, believe it or not, it's Jake!"

"Jake? He is a baby. Where in the hell, oh, never mind, tell me about it."

"Well, I agreed to take him to the mall with his friends, heck might as well I thought, no one will let him skateboard anywhere around here."

"Yeah, go on," I encouraged her and leaned forward over the phone.

"So when we get there, I thought it was weird but he wanted to take his book bag from school. So I stopped him and told him to get back in the car asking him why he needed his book bag since he never studies or uses it at home. So he says in his usual abundant vocabulary, 'I dunno.' So I said, 'Open it, what's in there?' As soon as that thing unzipped, I could smell it!"

Kidding her I said, "Gee, Jackie, how did you know what it was?"

"Ah, I went to school with Clinton, he wasn't the only one that did not inhale. I swear to God, I wanted to kill Jake and laugh at the same time. I didn't know what to do! So I took his book bag, and at the same time fearing that if he got near me I might have to hurt him! I told him I expected to see him home at five o'clock sharp. So he comes home with his friends and we talk. By this time, of course, his father is home and we are half-tempted to smoke the stuff ourselves! No, just kidding. We sit him down at the table and Jake says he has never smoked it before, but I don't believe him. Now I know why his grades have been in the toilet and he eats me out of house and home. I just thought he was growing fast! So I, like, do the parent thing and take him to the hospital and ask for a drug test to see if he would confess. Can you believe it? They told me I need his permission to test him!" Jackie exclaimed.

"Nothing surprises me anymore," I responded.

"What should I do?" Jackie asked.

"Smoke the stuff, find out if it is any good, then tell him to have his connection deliver to the house!" I laughed.

"You're real funny Allie."

"Hey, that extra money we were trying to make this summer, do you think we could grow it? Did you notice any seeds?" I teased her.

"Allie, neither one of your girls were stupid enough to get caught if they were doing it. Denial is great, I really just want to pretend that nothing ever happened. I felt dumb at the hospital, but I also feel like I have to do something," Jackie pleaded for an answer.

"Well, the first thing," I said in a more serious tone, "is the friends have to go. The grades have to come up, the clothes have to change. What else does he like?"

"His skateboard," Jackie answered.

"Well, that needs to be limited use to where you can watch him. He blew the trust, now he has to earn it back. Make him do a research paper on pot; what it is, what it does, what the consequences are if he had gotten caught by someone besides Mom! If you really want to stir up the pot, pardon the pun, call the mothers of the kids that you took to the mall with you," I told her.

"I couldn't do that Allie, do you really think I should?"

"Would you call me if it had been one of my girls?" I asked.

"Yeah, but I can talk to you. You know how I am, but these mothers don't. What if their kids had nothing to do with it?" Jackie asked hesitantly.

"Then they know your little brat is the troublemaker," I harassed her with the truth.

"You are so very funny, Allie, real funny. I think you need to adopt a twelve-year-old boy to understand," Jackie warned.

"You know Jackie, it's his choice, it's his mistake, it's his challenge. If you ever want to bring him down here to the clinic for the day, you know that would be an education in itself," I told her seriously.

"You know I am just fit-to-be-tied, Allie," she said.

"Well, we both were before this happened!" I said. "He is just going to force you to be more active in the parenting thing. Like, he got the fun and you get punished, I know. But better this way than the cop calling you from the police station or school letting you know he just got kicked-out or worse, arrested! What did you do with the stuff?"

"We flushed it down the toilet in front of him. Neither one of us have seen that stuff since college. Ahh, the benefits of an education..." Jackie's voice trailed off.

"Shame on you mom, at least you can laugh again. It is serious but it's out in the open now and not going anywhere, it has to go back on him. Just make sure he understands the consequences and you might want to work out something with the counselor and teachers, just for the team effort. Since he most likely scored it on the playground, you might ask some questions. This is the age when they make it or break it," I said trying not to scare her. "Still going to do dinner with me tomorrow?"

"Sure, Allie, I need to take a break," she assured me.

"Hang in there mom, it will be okay," I tried to reassure her.

"Thanks Allie, I knew you would at least make me laugh. See ya tomorrow," and Jackie hung-up the phone.

"Damn, that is too close to home," I said under my breath. Then I thought *sixth grade upper-middle class neighborhood, gosh and golly, so much for the D.A.R.E. program.*

"Hey, Jack, you busy?" I asked him over the intercom.

"No, darling, anything for you," he crooned.

"Are you going to the federal thing that you do tonight?"

"Yes, ma'am, got a television there to watch the game while I collect piss samples, even bought a fresh cigar for the night." Jack stated.

"Do you have access to a couple of extra test kits? My girlfriend just busted her kid with pot. Is it true that a parent cannot force their kid to drug test?" I asked him because I knew he knew all the answers.

"Yes, ma'am. Those little potheads have rights," he told me.

"Well, get me a couple of kits, okay?" I asked him.

"I have some here with me now, I'll be right over with them," he said. Good ole' Jack, always ready for anything.

~ ~ ~

"Allie, Curly is here to see you," Ethel announced on the speakerphone.

"Okay, Ethel. I am going to come down, she can dose and I'll meet her out front," I told her.

I remembered the first time I met Curly. I gave her that name because when I first saw her she was huddled in a ball on the outside steps and all you could see was a mass of dirty blondish curls. Jack told Moses to come and get me because it was my turn to do rescue.

"My turn for what?" I asked Moses.

"To sit with this young lady," he said.

I asked, "Who is this?"

"We don't know but she found our stairs and has used just a little too much of something, doesn't smell like liquor though. We are trying to keep her conscious," said Moses.

"Does Doc know?" I asked him.

"Yeah, Jack, Doc, and myself figured this is the best solution. She is a little better than before, see if you can get her name. And Allie, don't touch her, she has been on the street for a while, okay?" Moses warned me. "Care with caution, just try to keep her talking and figure out what she is taking. We couldn't find any tracks on her arm."

"Sure, Moses," I reassured him as I went to the front stairs.

So, I attempted to converse with a malnourished, dirty, barefoot, childlike woman who was trying to curl into the fetal position. I started with, "Hi, I am Allie."

She lifted her head slightly, her eyes roll, her head drops back down, and a soft mumble came from her mouth. Someone had used her for a punching bag too.

"Come on sweetie, try to sit up and lean against the stairs. Come on, we have to keep your head up. Do you live around here?" I asked as I attempted to sit her upright.

Another mumble came from her lips.

"What is your name?" I encouraged in my most compassionate tone.

Again, only a mumbling sound was given as an answer.

"What did you take?" I ask. "This is a safe place, you can tell us, we want to help you. She cried almost a giggle, then more mumbles. She was beaten-up pretty bad, cuts and bruises on her legs and arms. I could not even tell when she might have last taken a bath. When she finally got her eyes to stay open in an attempt to focus, I could see they were a beautiful shade of blue. As I sat there looking at her, my mind started to wander *What made her come here? What has she seen, or been through? Does anyone care that she is still alive?*

Then I said, "Hey, Curly, do you have family we can call?" No shoes, no purse, obviously no identification. She was in shorts and a blouse that may have looked nice at one time. In fact, *she* may have looked nice at one time. "Curly, where do you live?"

She mumbled again.

"Can I get you some water?" I still tried to reach her.

"Sure, that would be nice," she finally responded.

Oh my God, we connected! I marched into the dispensing area and got her a cup of water. "She lives!" I announced. I brought her back the water, but she was gone.

That was the way it went around here. It was several weeks before we saw Curly again. Of course, she had no recollection of our initial encounter. Jack gave her the "you scared the hell out of us" routine and how bad it would be for business if she decided to die in front of our clinic. The least she could do was get on the program before she ruined our reputation around town.

I noticed this time, Curly was slightly cleaner, but obviously still living on the streets without anyone. I guess she was a working girl and not doing such a good job at it. She eventually settled in at the Christian shelter down the street. They had given her some medical attention and got her cleaned up. After that, she looked almost nice some of the time. The poor kid really needed a dentist though. She had many broken teeth and they looked like they hurt.

"Curly, what's happening?" I asked her.

"I wanted to ask you for a transfer," she stated.

"Where are you going? You can't leave us now," I said.

"I got me an ole' man and we are going to San Diego," Curly flatly stated.

"Hey, the beach, that sounds better than here," I tried to sound encouraging.

"I guess," she said.

"What do you mean, I guess?"

"Well, you know, I still gotta work and all," she lowered her head.

"Well, you don't have to go. You can stay at the home can't you?" I asked trying to encourage other options.

"No, the pastor found out we had been seeing each other which broke his stupid rule, so we have to leave. That's the only reason we are going to San Diego. My ole' man has some family there he said, and hell, I ain't got nothing here," she said sounding more depressed.

"So, do you know which clinic you are going to there?" I asked her.

"No, they said you could get me a list."

"Sure, no problem," I told her and got the information. I printed a list of the clinics in that area and handed it to her. But as far as I know, she did not call for a courtesy dose or a transfer within the allowed fourteen days.

Jack's fear was that the asshole ole' man probably sold her to some "snuff" filmmaker south of the border. When he explained to me what that was, it made sense. We were most likely the only ones who would miss her. It made me sick when Jack joked about the girl making it into the movies, but she had to die to be a star. Things like this really scared the hell out of me. Especially when I thought about my own girls, my friend's girls, even my girl clients. The other issue Curly's case brought up was the date-rape drug which was most likely what Curly had been given, including a few others no doubt. Then someone dumped her on our doorsteps, she sure as hell could not have walked here on her own. At this clinic, we witnessed such a sad part of our world.

~ ~ ~

"Harry, what is that thing on your arm?" I asked one of my clients.

"What's it look like to you, Allie?" he asked right back.

"How long have you had it?" I asked him.

"It popped-up yesterday, worst damn thing I ever got. I guess I got some of that bad stuff that's going around. You know, I am really sort of scared. You hear of that flesh-eating disease on the news, did you?" he asked with real concern.

"Sure I have," I said. "Why don't we go see Doc, okay?"

"Sure, how about tomorrow?" Harry asked.

"Nope, now, Harry," I insisted.

"Okay Allie, I don't really feel good. This is different from any abscess I have ever had before," Harry said as he walked with me down the corridor to Doc's office.

"Allie, this man needs to go to the hospital now!" Doc told me. "Not tomorrow, not tonight, now."

"Did you hear that Harry? Not tomorrow, not tonight, now. Do you want me to call someone?" I pleaded for him to say yes.

"No, I'll go," he tried to promise me.

"I'll call the hospital and let them know you are coming, you go, now. Did you dose?" the doctor asked him.

"Yeah, Doc," Harry replied.

"You go hospital right now, serious okay?" Doc made his plea to Harry.

"Okay, Doc, thanks," he said and left.

Harry died that night, I mean he became a fourteen day no show, but we all knew what had happened to Harry.

There was some pretty bad stuff going around. Everyone that was actively using had gotten some bad abscesses, one girl lost half her shoulder. I do not think it was the flesh-eating bacteria, but instead a blood infection that worked fast. The clients all asked for dose increases and left the dope alone for a while. Anyway, it was getting close to the holidays and they needed money for other things.

I remember the first time I witnessed how abscesses were treated. A sweetheart of a girl came back in bad shape after she had surrendered her power to everyone and ditched in a hotel room with a bag of dope for a week. She went to the doctor across the street and I casually walked over to check on her. The doctor asked me to help hold her down while they packed the abscess. First, it must be opened and cleaned. It was like the worst looking giant hot three-inch pimple you have ever seen, boiling red in color with heat radiating off it. Next, the doctor lanced and drained it, then cleaned it again and stuffed it with gauze. That poor girl left bruises on my arm from holding on so tight. I had to focus directly into her eyes; I did not handle it too well.

It did not take a urine test to figure some things out. We heard stories from the clients with the insider's knowledge about the chemicals used to make some of the intoxicants. These people knew that sometimes there was even cut glass in the stuff they used. One guy told me he watched as jet fuel was being used in Mexico to cut speed! We even heard about children using cleaning fluid to get high! This was just some of what was really going on.

At these times, Jack and I would get into our debates over legalization of drugs. "It should all be destroyed and every pusher locked-up," he and Angie would rant.

It will never go away I thought to myself.

From the beginning of time, man has found ways to alter his consciousness, to break the mundane of normal existence. How *could* it just end? Look at how far beer dates back—I read that the trails of the pilgrims were altered because of beer rations! My thoughts keep piercing my brain *You don't see kids selling beer on the playground, maybe it should be legal! You don't hear about killings in other countries over drug wars, is it news censorship, or does legalization work?*

I decided it all boiled down to profit, world economy, and employment. Many jobs were created within drug trafficking, not just heroin, but all the drugs. So why curb it?

~ ~ ~

"Jack, I have a weird situation here. My client says he called in yesterday, Sunday, for a no show excuse. He stopped me this morning to see if it messed up his chance at getting a take-home, but the dispensing record says he was here. He says he was not. What the heck do I do with this?" I asked with sincere concern.

"Well, Allie, it all depends, how honest are you? I sure wouldn't let someone make a profit if they didn't share," Jack said with a hint of sarcasm in his voice.

"What do you mean?" I asked, not understanding his innuendo.

"Do you have any idea what one 80 milligram dose on the street goes for these days?" Jack asked.

"Gee, no Jack, guess it's not on my shopping list," I teased.

"Well, let's just say in some areas someone could get an easy one hundred for pocket money," he stated flatly.

"For one dose?" I naively asked.

Jack then explained the game to me, "The nurse is the one that takes all the calls. The doctor is not around, Javier is not around, so who monitors the phone calls? The client doesn't care, it just looks like he is here, and who the hell is going to believe the client anyway? So, like the client calls, the nurse delivers the dose to her pocket and no one notices a few doses missing because most clients won't question it and *voilà*! The weekend nurse has a nice cash business."

"So, what do I do about this?" I asked in disbelief.

"It is up to you, as I said, I wouldn't let someone make a profit without sharing!"

"Gee, thanks Jack. You are a big help!" I hung-up the phone.

I went down to dispensing and told the head nurse of my dilemma. She responded, "I'll look into this and tell Javier."

The next thing I heard on this topic was that the clinic was looking for a new nurse for the weekend shift. Apparently, this had been going on for some time. The clients knew about it, it was just the first time one of them came to a counselor and the Director had something concrete to work with for action to take place. It made me wonder just how long this little scam had really been going on.

~ ~ ~

"I am really getting burned-out with southern California," I told my friend Jackie. "I am sick of the traffic, I am sick of the crime, I am sick of the news. I hate the heat and the smog. I am just sick and tired of being sick and tired."

"Why do you stay?" Jackie asked.

"Where do I go?" I said.

"I know Allie, I feel the same way and with what happened with Jake we recently put the house up for sale and we have an offer on it already. We didn't even get the sign up and it was sold! You know John has been interviewing all over the country and we were only supposed to be located here for two years and it's already been seven. So when this happened the other night with Jake and the pot, John was in the middle of trying to negotiate a better offer, but then he said, 'That does it, we are out of here.' Since the day I arrived here, I have hated this place," Jackie told me.

"I know what you mean and you live in a much better area than I do! Who will I complain to when you leave, and where the hell are you going to go?" I asked.

"Where we moved from, Washington. I am going to be gone for a couple of weeks house hunting. John's new employer is going to pay most of the moving expenses and part of the escrow," she said.

"I am going to miss you, Jackie, can I come visit?" I asked eagerly.

"Sure you can, you know our girls will keep in touch. I am going to miss the stories from the clinic," Jackie said clearing her throat of emotion.

One of my few friends in this town was leaving me. So much for our lavender farm, another dream of our escape together.

"Write me, Allie," she said.

"Sure, Jackie, sure," I droned with sadness.

Now, Mom was gone and my girls were now out of the house. Jackie would soon be gone and my husband I actually wished was gone! Jack was also being weird for the past several weeks. Everyone was doing something different but me. I told myself I would get out of this town when the girls were out on their own. Well, I decided to put the house up for sale, just to see what happens. A fight ensued about putting the house up for sale, it was harsh. My beloved partner, albeit currently estranged, who had agreed ten years earlier to our plan of escaping to Mexico, called me an "unrealistic fool."

Well, I will show him! I thought to myself.

My sister and I took Thanksgiving weekend to go up the coast to explore where I could settle if the house sold. We found a house to rent in a beautiful little coastal town that was just what I had envisioned, it felt right. I asked the owner to keep me in mind and filled out the application. I told her I would call when I had a better idea of when my escrow would close. When I returned home there was an offer on my house. My idea of freedom was becoming real at last! I accepted the offer on the house; they wanted to move in before Christmas.

20 A Search for Freedom

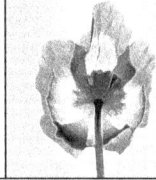

Christmas at the clinic always started before Thanksgiving. The clients had to test clean for the holiday take-homes and that could be anytime from Thanksgiving weekend on. The staff always planned the annual holiday party for the clients. We had plenty of free toys to wrap up for the kids, thanks to Angie. And there was the great food, lots of excuses to have fun at work!

Last year, Jack and I volunteered to do the food, we were going to show them how to do it right. We bought expensive coffee and bagels with a variety of toppings, fresh juice and fruit. We had an entire day off with pay to go shopping. We managed to do it in one hour and one stop, Jack had to get to the track of course. The leftover bagels were enough for the entire year and the clients got plenty of the "good stuff" coffee.

Needless to say, we did not have to worry about the party this year and it was a good thing, Jack was stuck in his asshole mode hiding in his office. Many of us were beginning to speculate that Jack had relapsed. The counselors came to me like I had the answer, but the truth was I had no idea why Jack was acting so weird. He had just quit talking. I said, "Maybe he is just tired." It seemed he was at war with one of the nurses and not getting along with anyone else. When Jack was at war, the clinic was not the same. Of course, now anything that happened out-of-line, Jack was suspect.

My estranged husband called to tell me he had just rented a house, I figured so much for the reconciliation efforts. I proceeded to speak with Javier and made a big decision in less than five minutes. I told him I was in financial straits, my house had sold, and I had a chance to move North by the beach. First, he asked if he could escape with me, then he offered a leave of absence. I now know I should have taken him up on the offer, but at the time, I told him it would not be fair to the clinic and I thought next week would be my last day.

The staff did not want me to leave. They did, however, find hope in my journey that someone could move forward. We all were in a rut at the clinic, not much different than the clients. We were trapped by the hours, the income, and the benefits. The most difficult task I had now was to inform the clients that I was leaving. Everyone in their lives had left them at one time or another. I reminded myself that my leaving was a good thing and that maybe some of them had become too dependent on my support. The truth was I had become dependent on them, however, I did not see this at the time. All I could see was getting to a place where there was no traffic, no special report due every hour; or, where I found myself glued to the television waiting for the picture or a name to see if it was one of my clients. I longed for serenity, quiet, and sleep. I had managed to secure employment through the Internet in the new location. I figured it would do until I could get acquainted with the neighborhood. After all, they must have heroin addicts where I was going, right?

Many of the clients just shut down when I told them I was leaving, some requested to be transferred to certain counselors. The staff gave me a good-bye lunch and a housewarming basket. I had one client break down and cry. She said, "It's Javier, isn't it?"

I said, "No, it is time for me to follow my own advice. How long have I told you to find a goal and follow your dream? Besides, I can't afford to stay here, so this is my chance. "

The day before my last day, this client went next door to find me and offered to give me money, not much, she just wanted to help me. It hurt and felt good at the same time. These were the people I worked so closely with, my clients. They had nothing, but gave everything they had.

~ ~ ~

The worst was yet to come, Eleanor was in the hospital. I did not call or go see her right away because I felt I was hiding information from her, like my clients did when they did not want me to know something. Now, it was time, I needed tell her of my move. I really did not have to, it is just who I am.

It was Friday and it had been raining hard for over a week. I cried for two days, I really was not aware of just how loved I had been. Leaving this group, the staff and the clients, was like leaving my home. I tried to find several excuses not to go to the hospital that day, but found myself sitting on the bed waiting for Eleanor to return from a medical test. It was the hardest thing I have ever done professionally, to say good-bye to Eleanor.

Of course, I promised all my clients they would get my address and that I would keep myself accessible to them. At the time, I did not know that Jack and Angie would not give them this information. It was just as well, the only news they would have shared with me no doubt would have been bad. So I drove home crying, stuck in traffic in the rain. No Christmas party, no clinic, no clients, no more family. I could not think about that, I had a house to pack up in less than forty-eight hours and then I would be off to discover my new life.

The rain finally stopped about forty-five miles before I reached my destination in northern California. I arrived about 10:00PM, the town was locked-up tight and looked like a postcard from the past. This was now my home. It was cold, the sky was full of stars which you could actually see, and I could hear the pounding of the surf and seabirds in the distance. It seemed to me at that moment, I had heard only one bird for years, the damn rooster from the clinic! Now, like music there was the sound of birds everywhere and the lush smell of flowers. It had been a long time since I smelled anything but clinic trash, dead rats, and urine.

I must admit, that first day was total chaos. Back home, I could find day-workers all the time on any corner, but here no one knew what I was talking about when I inquired about hiring a few men to help me unpack my truck. Luckily, I found two students that had formed their own moving company. They were just getting ready to hit the beach when I called. Where I had paid five dollars per hour to load the truck, I was asked to pay sixty dollars per hour to unload it! They were, however, kind enough to give me a ride home after the truck was unloaded and dropped off at the rental return site.

I questioned these young men about the kids in the area. They reported, "No, no real drug problems around here. No, no gangs. No, not many problems except bad wave sets."

Of course, this was a coincidence I thought; these kids must just be the "good kids." There are a few left, right? Checking out my new town, I saw no writing on the walls, no baggy pants, and I did not see one person wearing slippers! I did not feel tension in the air and the town only had 2800 residents, so there was no traffic. I knew I had landed in paradise.

I had two weeks to unpack and get acquainted with the town before I was to start my new job. I had never been so alone in my life. I was so caught up in the move that the reality of Christmas escaped me, it was in three days. I could not find a tree anywhere. My girls came up to see me and it was weird and a bit unsettling. We had gifts around a poinsettia plant which was the closest thing to a tree I could find. I burnt the turkey, as well as, my hand and it was all just a nightmare. Later, every time I looked at that burn scar, I saw a healing abscess. Jack and

Moses got online and we communicated by email. They both commented that only I could mistake a burn for an abscess and that it was not a good enough excuse for me to get out of my new job. They also wrote that the clinic had found someone to take my caseload and to enjoy my new life. My daughters could not understand why I was sad, this was my *dream* they reminded me.

~ ~ ~

I slept a lot the first week and I stayed up late. I became reacquainted with network television, as well as, other things I had abandoned years ago due to my clinic hours. A few mornings my internal clock forced me out of bed and I laughed as I watched the early morning traffic report. I giggled that just a few weeks ago, I would have been the one stuck in that traffic jam!

I kept reminding myself that this was the right thing to do and the right place to be. I started to walk in the mornings, there were people walking everywhere. It was so peaceful, beautiful, and quiet, except for the birds which sounded like continual music to me.

I showed up early for the first day of my new job, the drive there was beautiful. I laughed to myself at the comparison of the California coastline with its green rolling hills scattered with cattle and deer compared to a congested freeway with uptight angry people. No traffic here. The only people out at this time in the morning were those jogging or walking their dogs. Whoopee!

The new employers explained there had been a change in my job due to my experience. I would still get the same compensation (like that was the only thing that mattered) but I was to do data entry. I guess this was the price to pay for something different.

I can do this I said to myself *I have arrived in paradise.*

Working with addicts was a breeze compared to working with the straight and sober. We had joked at the clinic about never fitting into the rest of society again, well, I was having a hard time. Now that I did not need to wake up in the middle of the night, I found I could not sleep through it. I began looking at everyone and tried to figure out what drug they were on! I certainly received mixed messages from people. I just knew these folks were sick, pretending to be healthy. Back at the clinic, at least the addicts knew who they were and did not try to be anything but authentic dope fiends.

The politics of the office, not to mention the noise level, was just too much. Eight hours a day of no communication and simply typing was just more than I could handle, I quit. I worked my new job a mere thirty days. It did not dawn on me until I talked to my sister and brother, who also quit their jobs on this same day, that it was the one-year anniversary of our mother's death.

The escrow on my house had fallen through but there was another offer made and it was going to close the end of the month. My estranged husband who did not think I would really move was now promising me the sun and moon if I would just come back. I started to doubt my decision.

Ignoring all of my obvious stressors like the death of my Mom, a pending divorce, my children leaving the nest, and a complete change of employment and environment, I began asking myself *Was I crazy selling the house? What am I doing here? Who am I?* No longer a wife, daughter, mother, counselor, or homeowner, I felt alone.

~ ~ ~

Angie from the clinic called to see how I was doing.

"I quit my job," I told her.

This excited her because the person they had hired was not working out and she insisted I come back to the clinic.

I did not know what to do, so I surfed the net, did some day-trading then walked along the beach. I listened to the birds, smelled the fresh air, and slept even more.

I did a lot of internal questioning and thinking *The house is technically still mine, right? Maybe my relationship did have something worth saving. I could have my job back, but should I even go there again?*

I heard myself say aloud, "Does the counselor need counseling?"

Live the dream, this is paradise I told myself.

Then I heard myself mumble, "Find a therapist!"

I completed two different résumés, filled out some county job applications, called on a few want-ads and even made an appointment. But I felt homesick, lost, and lonely. I went to the movies by myself, joined an exercise class, and started to wander around where the locals did. There was nothing about this little town I could not celebrate.

The new therapist told me I had just gone through several of the most significant stressors one could experience in their life, and I did it all in one year! She suggested I just rest and have some fun. *Fun! What a concept!* I thought.

I connected with a methadone advocacy group that stated they had employment potential for the future. They were anticipating changes in the laws and were looking for someone to lobby for a change in the methadone arena. I was curious, it sounded like a great opportunity. I could use my experience for something, maybe travel and continue to work with this population. They invited me to a meeting in Washington, DC so I took them up on the offer.

I drove back down the coast in an effort to close the escrow on my house but was too afraid to stop at the clinic. While I was away, Ethel had left a message on my machine, "Allie, we need to talk to you, it's Jack."

Of course, I immediately called back.

They all passed the phone around, it was nice to know I could always call the clinic at ungodly hours of the morning and find company. They talked about Jack and how he needed to take a road trip. So, when he got on the phone and stated he needed a session with his favorite counselor, I said, "Come on up!"

Jack asked if it would be okay to visit in two weeks. I told him, "Sure, that will give me time to go to Washington, DC and then we will have something to talk about besides the birds and the view from my living room." It was a date.

I also talked to Javier about the invite from this organization which I had come to know through the Internet. He did not know of the group but was aware of the big meeting in Washington, DC, so I committed to myself to attend. My plane ticket was going to be waiting for me at the counter.

I was alone, bored, and what-the-heck, it could turn into a job; besides, I had never been to Washington, DC. Of course, my estranged husband whom I left my dog with thought I was going to meet some axe-murderer that I had been having an affair with online. Actually, I had been communicating with just one individual who lived in a southern state. This was new federal grant money they were working with and it was just getting organized. Everything he told me I had been able to verify. He did not sound like an axe-murderer but he did not sound like a client either. As far as men were concerned, I just was not interested. I knew better.

Much to my surprise, not only this Internet person was a client, but the entire organization was comprised of methadone clients! They did not know at first that I was not on a program. I was taken by surprise, but so were they. I know that addicts can work and hold down jobs, but what I was not prepared for was this reverse prejudice. I ended up being one of the bad guys. I began to hear the tales of methadone nightmares from four different people living within four different states.

The gentleman who recruited me was currently driving two hours to get to his clinic for his dose. He was passionately involved with changing the laws. He wanted to know why he could not go to his doctor for treatment and get the prescription filled at the local pharmacy. I heard about the abuses of treatment and the different level doses. I could not believe the dose levels that were being given. Everyone had a story and a theory.

All this talk reminded me of one lady on my caseload who had been prescribed methadone for a stomach disorder. I did not follow up on her story but our doctor never really believed it. I learned several doctors had prescribed methadone for a variety of reasons, but then the patients ended up needing to go to a clinic for treatment where they were treated like scum. Who could blame them for being upset and wanting to make legal changes?

What an education I received at that conference. It was the opposite end of the war on drugs, it was the lobby to legalize and liberalize. I met some very passionate and educated advocates and health professionals. Seminars were held hourly for people from all over the world working together to bring the war on drugs to an end. They showed innovative ideas from Europe on outreach; just imagine, drug warnings on clothing tags for young girls!

I saw information and workshops on the methods of getting the word out about AIDS, safe-sex educational programs, and of course, the facts and figures on the war on drugs were everywhere. At every booth I also found out about the difficulties in distributing all these facts to the public.

I heard talks on the privatizations of prisons and the fastest rising companies besides Internet stocks. I read brochures on the discriminatory facts toward Blacks and Hispanics and how dozens within these groups were getting pulled over by law enforcement for no reason. I read statistics like one out of every three Black men end up in prison. This literature discussed places like Baltimore, where there was a lower ratio of men to women because of this occurrence and the difficulty of having positive male role models for their youth in that city. The facts on the moneymaking end of things was also addressed, like entire budgets being slashed to encourage the police to confiscate more property, guilty or not.

The mayor of San Francisco attended the conference also, boasting of his innovative programs. Several well-known drug rehabilitation educators and researchers were also there. The most impressive was a policeman from Canada who decided to "out himself" as a pro-legalization supporter. Were these people the "Lindas" of the world who had decided to fight the system the right way? It was truly an education for me to be in attendance at that conference.

The smell of pot in the hallways was startling! I mean usually you get asked "smoking or nonsmoking" in motels and as you walk through the lobbies you smell the lingering odor of cigarette smoke. However, I think one could have gotten a better contact-high walking through the halls on the seventh floor of this motel than any Jimmy Buffet concert! Of course, I am sure most of it was for prescription use. Do not misunderstand me, these were important people. Many had done a lot in the way of drug rehabilitation and educational outreach. These were people who *knew* there was something else going on.

The women attending the conference reminded me of many of my precious clients; the clubbed hands from heroin use, the medical complications that go with this population, and the attitude. In one group, all the women had been diagnosed with the Hepatitis C virus and were angry that the information regarding treatment was not readily available. They were fearful of the future and how they would get their dose.

One gentleman I met had never used heroin, so he said. He stated that his doctor had prescribed methadone for him like they did Ritalin for children. He took 60 milligrams in the morning and 60 milligrams twelve hours later. This dose, to me, was hard to imagine but he said his wife refused to live with him without it. I never saw him nod-off or miss-a-beat and he was incredibly articulate.

For too many of those in attendance, the handicap of methadone controlled their lives, yet they had lives because of methadone. Most could not get past the fact that I was from the "other side." They clearly wanted me to know they had been abused by the systems beyond my charm and sincerity. To be honest, I did not know if I could support their agendas.

Sure there were special circumstances, it is like kids and sex. Do you teach abstinence or hand out condoms? This was the hand out condoms group. Do you give out clean needles or do you force everyone to take Naltrexone (a drug which decreases the craving for narcotics and alcohol) like Jack suggested?

While I was there, I was able to review the details of some of the programs in different states and countries. I noticed where some of my ideas like active listening to each client, being truthful and open, as well as, my holistic views were actually being put into action and even working! These programs also took a lot of money. I still think if someone took the time to help with the psychological dependence, many people would not need to use methadone for the rest of their lives. However, many professionals are, or have been, convinced this system of methadone treatment to halt heroine use is the only way. Does a diabetic always have to continue using medication (insulin), if he changes his diet, exercises, and ultimately stabilizes his sugar? No. Can methadone be used in this same manner? I thought so.

I remembered my mother panicking at the dose taper her doctor had suggested after months of using a cortisone drug. She was afraid because it helped her breathe, or so she thought. Sure she had side effects from it but she learned to live with them. She was completely freaked out about this drug not being in her system. To me this seemed no different than what my clients felt when facing methadone detoxification; panic and fear of the unknown, but then came acceptance and stability.

~ ~ ~

We missed the bus that went to the lobby on Capitol Hill due to some confusion. I was glad because I was not completely sure where I stood on certain issues. I took what information I felt important and flew home. I am still stuck on the issue of physicians prescribing methadone. I do not understand why some of the HMOs and PPOs have not taken this one on. It would be an inexpensive endeavor since most of the big medical programs already offer Chemical Dependency Clinics, as well as, behavioral health policies. There would be better medical management and they could possibly offer more affordable treatment. In addition, the client could receive uninterrupted treatment within this model. Since there are other medications clients must take for the rest of their lives, even codeine; why wouldn't this setup work with methadone?

Is the problem with the ignorance surrounding the methadone itself? Is it the population of those people receiving it? If it is the population, why is there not a Drug Dealer Program something like the program for sex offenders? The methadone client would just need to register and report. The Probation Department could give out the dose and see the individual every day. There are solutions, some could be simple solutions.

I began thinking to myself that maybe the problem was a belief in the impossibility of rehabilitation. Or, maybe it was the amount of personal effort required by a physician that methadone requires? I knew so many clients that would benefit from being away from the clinic life. They needed to completely lose the identity which they came to the clinic in the first place to shed. I asked myself *Do the systems that control our country's poor and addicted, really want things to change?*

Upton Sinclair, a noted author (born in 1878, died in 1968) was a believer in social reform and being honest with the American people. He was a proclaimed alcoholic with political and social ideals which included helping those in poverty and in need of social reform. One of Sinclair's famous quotes answers my question, "It is difficult to get a man to understand something when his salary depends on his not understanding it." *This* is part of what is going on.

On my flight home from DC I continued my thinking—*I sure wouldn't mind doing counseling in a nice office close to the southern California coastline. It would be a good place for rehabilitation, better than the jungles of LA County. Well, this probably won't happen, at least not soon.*

21 | Questioning Our View

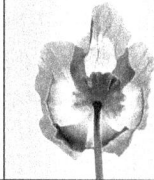

I came back to the birds, the beach, and unemployment. Jack called to confirm his reservation at Allie's Beach Resort.

I said, "Yeah, but don't expect room service." He laughed and said he always knew I was too smart to take one of his checks.

Jack and I were really like brother and sister. One does not spend seven to eight hours a day with others and not develop some sort of relationship. All of us at the clinic, despite the sibling rivalries, the BS of the job, and intermittent contempt for Javier, were a perfect dysfunctional family.

We all had our problems including Davey's new marriage and baby; Angie's eating disorder; Bonnie's family situation which by now must include two grandchildren and two daughters-in-law; Todd's cancer which was a big nightmare; and, Javier's separation from his wife. The clinic staff provided the nurturing for one another which was lacking from our own homes.

I missed my clients and all their questions: "Is so-and-so clean?" "What happened on so-and-so's drug bust?" "How is Eleanor?" I saw my clients every day, like a family too. I did not spend a great deal of time with them but I did talk to them every day. It was like checking the mood of my kids before they went to school. The chance to get into their mind was fascinating to me, to be allowed to go where no one had been allowed to go. Also, the chance to make a difference in someone's life meant a great deal to me. God, how I missed it!

Teaching, coaching, learning, everything else seemed so trivial now. How could I sit and type when I might be able to remind a man that despite his past, he was still a father and husband? Or to remind a woman that just because she used heroin, she was still a mother and a role model for her children. Who would point out their other choices, the ones they did not think about? Who would tell them that today was over but there *is* a tomorrow? Or that relapse was okay because it shows you how far you have come and what you stand to lose if you choose to go back to old habits. Who would tell them that someone may have given them the label of "addict" which they were wearing, but I thought they were a miracle waiting to happen? Who would ask them, how does being an addict serve you? And who was going to tell them to drink more water for gosh-sakes?

Jack pulled up about two hours later than he estimated and I had to make a shopping-run. So, as soon as he put his bag down, I got him in the car and off we went. He asked me, "What's the big deal about moving so far? The stores all look the same once you get inside!" As we were driving, he pointed and asked, "What's that?"

I said, "The men's prison."

"What's that?" he repeated.

I said, "A deer."

"No wonder you like it up here, the men are in cages and the animals roam free!" he said.

"Yep, you got it," I said. "Now, behave yourself. I have connections with the guard at the gate!"

So the conversation was light but I could tell he was nervous. We agreed to go to dinner while we were out. He could not believe how the town shut down at 8:00PM sharp. We had a great dinner and he alluded to talking afterward. He kept building on a story without saying a word, like a tourist who keeps asking questions about a town.

"How much longer are you going to stay on vacation?" he finally asked me.

"Do you mind if I get a bottle of wine? I prefer my fiction with a little alcohol," I teased him.

"Make it two!" he laughed.

I bought him a bottle of nonalcoholic beer. He sat down next to the door when we returned home. So he could jump out before I tossed him out, he said. He then began to unravel his story. "It's my 'I am God' complex," he said.

Jack and I had shared dreams of doing a private counseling thing together so he thought he would start his new practice with his friend's daughter as his first client, but he forgot he was human. He forgot about all the rules of AA, like a man cannot sponsor a woman or a woman sponsor a man. He forgot his ethics, he forgot about needing distance between personal and professional issues. Jack had a personal attachment to the outcome, like he said he got confused with his

"I am God" syndrome.

He continued telling me he had known this girl's family since she was little. He knew her parents and was a friend of the family. After years of listening to Jack's BS, I still could not tell his fiction from fact. I looked at him funny and started chewing off my artificial nails. Since there was nowhere around I could afford to get them filled, they were not needed in my new life.

Jack told me about this girl and how it all started when he went over to tell her family about his mom who has been in a nursing home for the last few months. I knew about this and figured the event was part of his personality change several weeks ago. Jack was the only son and had a relationship with his mom like my brother had with ours. He lived alone and had no children, so most of his mother's care fell on his shoulders.

According to Jack, this girl had been trouble since she hit adolescence. She had been arrested when she was in her late teens or early twenties, he could not remember. The police officer apparently had not taken much information and she had plastic cuffs on which were easy for her to remove. So, when he left her sitting in the car, she escaped. She had managed to hide in the bushes without being found, then made her way home.

When she arrived home, she confessed her dilemma to her mother and convinced her to take her out-of-state to an aunt's house. The mother took her daughter's tennis shoes, which were caked with mud, out to the garage while the girl changed clothes and showered before the quick departure. Then the girl's father came home and after hearing the story agreed with the mom and offered to drive his daughter to the aunt's home. However, the father took her directly to the police station instead!

It took awhile for the mother to catch-on but one night she followed her husband out to the garage and found him clutching their daughter's dirty shoes and crying. He knew he had done the right thing but the pain of his choice was more than he could bear. He just kept clutching the tennis shoes.

"Good story, huh Allie?" Jack took a breath.

"Yeah, Jack. Cut the BS and get on with it," I reported back.

"Well, she got kicked-out of the aunt's house, and you know me, I am always telling people they can stay on my couch. I know I am obnoxious, that's why no one has ever taken me up on the offer. Anyway, late one night I thought one of the cats wanted the litter box changed but it was someone knocking at the door. It was early in November."

This is the same time Jack started acting so weird I thought to myself.

"So I let her in," he continued, "and I told her if she didn't bother me that she could sleep on the couch. She was actively using everything. My counseling so far had accomplished nothing. I know I started out right, I made up a treatment plan for her and everything. I told her where she could get a job, I even lined it up for her. I took care that she knew which buses to catch and told her she could stay at my place until she saved enough money to move out. Do you remember her? Her name is Stella, she has been on the program before."

"On the program? Have you totally lost your mind?" I screamed.

"Do you want me to leave?" he asked.

"No, go ahead and tell me this has a happy ending," I calmed down.

"Not yet, but I am working on it. First, it gets worse," he said lowering his head.

"I don't remember her face but the name sounds familiar," I said.

"So, she is working a job and back on the program," he explained.

"Please don't tell me that she is on your caseload!" I said afraid to ask.

"I really do make a mess of things when I decide to make a mess, don't I?" Jack asked in a *please don't hate me* tone.

"You mean all your questions about how I detoxed my patients was you garnishing information for her? You tried to rehab someone you are having an affair with?" I screamed as I removed all ten nails and drank half the bottle of wine.

"Now I can't get her to leave and she is still using. Allie, what do I do?" he begged.

I told him that his story was more drama than I had experienced in several weeks of television and I would see him in the morning. I told myself *this story cannot be true.* I suggested this to him over coffee the next morning.

Jack was punishing himself, he knew he had made a big mistake. I told him he should know better than to try to rescue someone. I also told him the reason she was still using was that he, like her parents (except for the story when her dad took her back to jail) kept rescuing her.

I asked him, "How many times have we gone over the phase 'You can lead a horse to water but sometimes he will just piss in the lake?' Like everything else at the clinic, confess your sin, get her off your caseload and give her a few bucks to get out of your apartment. How many times did you tell me, Jack, that 'the party is not over until the partier is done.' You have told me yourself that you sent people out to use just to have them realize how *done* they really were, or were not. Why didn't you just take on more work? Go to a meeting Jack," I told him hopelessly.

So he did. Jack even moved into a sober-living home, he also managed it. I guess he could not make Stella move, so he did instead. He quit the clinic to do outreach in one of the worst parts of California, this was typical of an addict's behavior. Confused by his actions which were obviously a type of punishment, he was looking for the abuse he thought he deserved.

I later asked Jack if he packed a weapon in his new digs and he said, "No, I would probably just hurt myself."

I asked him if it was one of those towns where they stop you at the city limits to check for weapons and if you do not have one, they give you one. He said it was but that he politely declined the weapon saying he just scored drugs off the local cops instead.

"You are so scary," I laughed.

I also asked Jack if he had relapsed but he avoided the question. He talked about how difficult it was to watch it all so close up again. At the clinic, we were never quite sure if the rumors about Jack were true or not. Supposedly, at one time he did get married but she had died of an overdose, or a drunken driving incident, or something terribly tragic. He certainly demonstrated classic shame-based behavior.

I had seen four counselors relapse in my time at the clinic, I never expected Jack to fall. I guess he was human after all. I still do not know for sure that he relapsed into his drug of choice, alcohol. I do not know how far down he went. We had discussed his temptations before but compromising his ethics may have been too much for him. Or, it may have been the "I can change her" syndrome.

We had talked many times about the human condition only rising to its weakest link. Perhaps, it was his own sobriety that Jack offered to me to save. And was it simply a confession of what he thought was his sin? I never truly believed Jack's story until I talked to Angie after he had quit. I never let on that I knew a thing. Someone at the clinic discovered his secret, Stella. She had take-homes and he collected her urine. I swear he did it on purpose, he crossed the line. He knew what he was doing, he made a choice.

After he left, Jack knew he could not get close to drugs and that he needed to stay away from old friends and old playgrounds. More questions ran through my mind—*So does that mean people in recovery should not be counselors? How long in recovery before you are recovered?*

~ ~ ~

Jack used to repeatedly say that he was an asshole, so what did we expect? I had heard it so often that one day when he got done with his "I am an asshole" routine, I shared my own little story with him.

"Look," I said, "I used to go around saying 'okay so I am a bitch, someday I will be the perfect bitch.' Then one day my husband pointed out to me that I had said it so many times, indeed I turned into one. He told me he thought I had perfected it! Maybe if I had not taken such pride in being a bitch, people would not think of me that way. Actually, Jack, you are an angel, my angel and an angel to others. You remind me how to laugh and have been my personal cheerleader. From now on, I want you to substitute the word *angel* for asshole!"

Before Jack left my little house on the beach, I reminded him of the things he had done for all the clients; the hope, the love and the acceptance he had shared and inspired. I told him to remember how he instilled the "power of the brain theory" in his clients. And also when and why I realized I did not accept the labels of "addict" or "alcoholic," they are way too limiting. Labels are such an excuse and our society benefits from people wearing them.

I reminded him of my client, Troy, and that he had "got it." Troy decided to *not* be an addict, and guess what? He was no longer one! And I reminded Jack about Roberto and how he figured out that the respect he finally received in looking different and having a job served him better than doing nothing but drink and get high. We did not make Roberto wrong or belittle him, so there was nothing for him to rebel against.

After Jack left, I soon began searching for my own clues to why I chose to be a counselor, and how I had initiated change in those I had worked with at the clinic. I remembered the women clients at the clinic and how they were starting to understand they could think for themselves and do for themselves. They were beginning to realize it was easier to struggle and win than to be a man's slave. By keeping their daughters in school as I had urged them to do, these women were starting to see a difference. So many cycles must be broken early in this population.

I kept thinking about the kids and how they seemed to be dumped at six weeks old in childcare because their parents were tired, angry, and frustrated with their cash flow. Then one of them is called "no good" because he cannot do his homework while bouncing around until all hours of the night with his parents in search of their favorite medication. Where does this boy go? He escapes into what is always there for him, *the life*.

My mind was on a roll as I thought about the girls. What about the girls? The daughter that hooks-up with the first guy that says "Hey, you're cute" because that is the first attention she has gotten from a man, or anyone in years. "There really *is* no mystery to the addiction game," I mumbled under my breath.

I decided to jot down a few of my thoughts and questions as they poured from my brain. When people get tired of paying for the reward of addiction at their children's expense, will they see the possibilities offered by the straight life? So much has to change within the systems. Maybe it was working with the kids at the prison that awakened me. That experience taught me that eighteen years of programming cannot be undone in a session or two of counseling. All those kids were there because no one cared. No one took the time to see their *possibilities* or guide them toward a *different direction.*

I remembered when I arrived at the clinic, I was told no one ever leaves the methadone program. Well, that is just not true and I proved it! I saw the possibilities within my clients and helped more than a few see them too. I learned I could not just tell them, they had to *feel* those possibilities. They had to *feel it to own it.* So how do we give people, children, a chance to own it? Where did we ever get the idea that addiction or being on methadone was an "incurable disease?" One day, did someone just see endless financial gain in keeping people addicted to methadone? Or is it a contrived evolution to weed out the weak? "No, no," I whispered to myself, "that can't be true!"

My mind could not stop as I searched for more answers to all my internal questions. Writing feverishly, I witnessed my thoughts. So what if someone did pot years ago, did it really make a difference now? What about money for after school sports versus metal detectors at the gates? And what is with all the commercials on television for medications/drugs? Not the "Just Say No" stuff but the pill to breathe easier, to have better sex, to end depression, to lower cholesterol, to stop nausea, to help you sleep, to gain weight, to lose weight, etc. We did get rid of the commercial ads for cigarettes and most hard liquor, but now we are told to take this or that pill to get slim, happy, and wise! How is this influencing our children?

Why can we have centers for weight loss on every corner supplying "legal speed" but cannot get a third methadone clinic in the state of Maine? Or the first one on Maui? Why can we not get over the "not in my backyard" syndrome? Society seems to be saying we should not trust our parents or our church, but here, take this pill and all will be well. What's really going on? I had never been tempted to use drugs even though many times I got asked, "So, what about heroin, don't you ever want to try it?"

"Hell no," I would say, "something that powerful scares me. Drugs are something you sell your soul for, I'll stick with something I can control, not that controls me."

What about helping people? Is that a disease? If I can sell someone on *life,* is this my calling, my purpose? Is counseling going to be my career choice? Is it a type of *codependence?* I hate that term, it is as bad as the word *dysfunctional.* They are buzzwords that like addiction. Many people have made a lot of money promoting them.

The studies researched which I applaud, can now photograph the brain at any time. It has been discovered that brain cells light up as much when a person is *obtaining* a drug, the score, as during the actual fix. So, do we need another pill to fix this? Most of the new treatments, even for quit smoking, require some sort of pill, patch, or counseling. "Whatever happened to plain willpower like Dad said?" I asked out loud, then realized I had been writing for hours.

~ ~ ~

In the middle of my mind-melt, Ethel called, "Do you want your job back because there is an opening?"

"Yes," I snapped with my head still whirling with answers to questions that would solve the world's problems. Inside, my rational self shouted *Are you crazy?*

Ethel said she would have Javier call me right away. Well, I knew how fast Javier did things so I went on the interview at the Real estate office in town anyway. Besides, the closest clinics to my new home were two hours away, and like my clients, I did not want to drive that far. I was the only one with a Real estate license who showed up and she needed someone right away. I did not have all the money for the necessary fees so I left saying I would call her back. I called back to the clinic. Javier was at a Director's meeting and to the best of Ethel's knowledge, now the job did not look good because the census was dropping again.

Soon it was June, I spent the last few months being autistic. Sitting alone in limbo I really *did* want to live, which was always a good sign. I needed to be around people, I needed meaning and purpose back in my life. I called the Real estate broker back and said, "I'll take the job." She loaned me the money to pay my fees.

I showed up for work the next day. If I had to sell Real estate to survive, I surely could do it there. However, as much as the area was paradise, with a population of 2800 there were not many houses for sale. I loved the little office but the other women there warned me, "This place is sick, be careful, it's contagious."

The office environment reminded me of what my therapist friend, Dora, once told me. She said the problem with my relationship with my husband was due to "graduate syndrome." She said after learning so many psychological theories, I had destroyed our communication lines which just made him feel insecure. Her words to me were, "You are diagnosing those in your life and that needs to be saved for clients only." Dora was right. I tried to stop talking about psychology and addiction altogether when I moved away. I thought I could leave the jargon behind me. It was not easy.

The Real estate office was great but the mother as employer and the daughter as employee left something to be desired. I now know why nepotism sucks; war, anger, frustration, and family crap does not belong at the office. The mother/employer was emotionally shutdown and a workaholic. The daughter was a drug addict and an alcoholic with a teenage son who was into pot and whatever else crossed his path. Well, I found myself counseling again, not selling real estate!

When my second husband and I first met and married, it was all so perfect. He was a Realtor and sold the properties, I took care of the mortgages. The change to my counseling profession and those terrible working hours at the clinic were the big factors which caused most of our domestic issues. Add in some of the physical changes like his diabetes diagnosis and my menopause and it spelled separation. We began talking again and I felt good about a possible reconciliation.

At that point, I was where I wanted to be, I knew it—I thought I knew it. I was truly living the dream. I had met some people, made a few friends and was having fun. My estranged husband had been in therapy now for almost eighteen months. He was changing. He was focused. He was relentless! The phone calls, the emails, the surprise visits, he was wearing me down. He wanted me back.

I did love where I lived, I loved my new friends, and I even enjoyed my work. But there was something missing: my family. I had been married more years of my life than not and it felt strange not to have my family near me.

Then my husband called me, "So, you are the counselor. You believe in recovery. Well, I am recovered! You preach family and commitment and you once committed to me. Well, I am here now for my woman!"

How could I say no? He had lost fifty pounds working-out, gotten his diabetes under control, reestablished his relations with his children, and made some new friends. All that was missing in his life was *me*. However, I wanted to live in my beautiful little town at the beach. I had made a connection with myself there. I was where I wanted to be, but… there is always a *but* isn't there?

I invited him up for the holidays.

My husband seemed like a new man. When he arrived, he demonstrated his new changes and his new relationship language. He talked about himself commuting the few hundred miles to work, but that really did not make sense to me. I felt if we were going to try to make our marriage work, we needed to live in the same house.

Then I was offered extra money to stay with the Realtor's office. I really wanted it all, the new job in the place I loved living and my husband back in my life. I turned the job down. I recommitted to my man who had jumped through every hoop I had placed before him. I gave my notice and agreed to move back home.

Paradise was beautiful but I had to give my marriage a chance or forever wonder, "Would it have worked if I had just moved back home?"

I sold everything and had my little house rented before I left. A few "going back home" parties with my new friends brought tears to my eyes. I still was not sure I was doing the right thing. I called Angie at the clinic just to give her my new phone number and address. I had been home in our new house with new furniture and a new puppy for only three weeks when the phone rang.

"Hi Javier, yeah, almost three weeks now. Work? No, I am not working. It is going okay but it's not the beach like up North. When do you need me?" I asked.

"Tomorrow, no, let's make it Monday, we need to break *the spouse* in easy," he instructed me.

Was it a counseling relapse? Was it an addiction? Was it the universe, or just that I was a born counselor? How could I effect change in the world, if I was not a player?

Besides, I am still trying to figure out what's really going on.

Epilogue

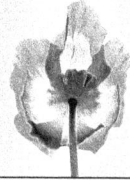

I have seen changes come about because of people becoming involved. It is these who are the real heroes in all this. Without
patient advocacy, changes will not come about within the present
system.

Dr. Vincent Dole

Deborah (Allie) continued to be one of the heroes who tried to find out
what is really going on within the field of addiction recovery. However,
Deborah would say it was her clients who were the real heroes and he-
roines. Interesting how the word *heroin* contains the word *hero*. She tried
to bring enlightenment to the addiction field while fighting her internal
battle over the clinical use of methadone versus cold turkey heroin detoxification.

Deborah moved away from the beauty and peace she had found near
the ocean in northern California to live among the traffic, smog, and fast-
paced city life of southern California once again. Because of her return to
working with those on methadone, as well as other substances, Deborah
directed hundreds of people to explore new directions and new possibilities for their lives.

Prior to Deborah's move North and then again when she returned to
southern California, I was living nearby and we would have our lunches
together to counsel and support one another about our personal relationships and, of course, to vent about the newest issues surrounding addiction
recovery. I am mentioned as Dora within this book. My private counseling

practice also surrounds the area of addiction and recovery and of the many areas of abuse which accompany this field. Deb and I both came from childhoods with an alcoholic parent. We shared the addiction background and the pain of having alcoholics within our families. We had a common desire to help unravel the mysteries of our clients and together continued questioning society's views on addiction.

Deborah and I also shared a passion to incorporate alternative and holistic therapies into the addiction arena. At one time, we developed a community of professionals in the surrounding area which would meet to discuss each other's dreams for expanding the circle of like-minded health professionals. We named the alternative healing group "Milagos" which means miracles in Spanish. When Deborah owned her Holistic Center, the members would meet every few weeks to explore and share our different professions. We agreed to develop our like-mindedness in holism by referring our clients/patients to one another. It was such fun to watch our community open to the many benefits of healing essential oils, acupuncture, massage, spiritual healing, counseling, and begin to educate themselves about the latest alternative techniques. Deborah and I began a new approach to wellness within that community which is still enjoyed today.

Within a year or so after her return from the northern California coastline, Deborah had an answer to her own marriage question of "Would it have worked if I had just moved back home?" She started divorce proceedings and moved near her beloved ocean once again, however, this time to the southern California coastline "…where it was a good place for rehabilitation." Because she did not move as far away this time, we could still meet for lunch as often as we could with the added distance between us.

I visited Deborah's little beach house in southern California and we walked arm an arm in the sand, again trying to solve the problems of the world. Deborah found peace living at the ocean for several years while working, playing, and learning that her chosen path of being a counselor was fulfilling her deep need to share her abundant compassion. She chose to continue working at clinics which served the addiction population, this was her passion.

Deborah had her two wonderful daughters visit when she needed to escape from the clinic's stress. They remember their mother just as I do, full of life and always being there for them and everyone else. Lisa, Deborah's younger daughter related to me that she wished she would have taken notes on how their mother raised her sister and herself. Lisa wrote, "I can remember how my Mom was *always* right about everything. It would drive me absolutely nuts, especially through my teenage years, because even at that time I knew she was right. She always gave us lots of freedom and she said it was because she trusted us. And because she put so much trust in me, I never wanted to let her down—a great parenting technique! I have so much appreciation for the way she guided us and shaped us to have big dreams and to instill the confidence it took to achieve them. I remember her always telling us... *I want you girls to spread your wings and fly.*"

In Deborah's amazing life she would make sure to tend to her friendships regularly. At one time, I introduced her to one of my favorite women, Becky Baker. Becky is also a substance abuse counselor whom I met at a time in my life when I needed counseling concerning alcohol use in my family and she provided just the right words of support. So the three of us, Deb, Becky, and I would meet for lunch and hash-out how we were going to survive the life of being a counselor. Our conversations could have gone on for days if we would have let them. Our voices and laughter could be heard throughout the restaurants, sometimes with glaring eyes; but no matter, we were solving the world's addiction problems!

Once, when I had an illness that stumped the medical profession, these two angels came to a "healing session" in my home to share their special energy. As I lie in bed with my Reiki Master working her magic, Deborah and Becky, as well as, one of my sisters (and many other soul-sisters not present) directed their healing energy into and through my body. This incredible experience was one of the most loving and spiritual events in which I have participated.

Deborah always supported my writing projects and attended my book signing events buying several copies for friends and clients. She would get off work and drive for hours just to attend and watch me sign my newest book. My willingness to help write and finish her extraordinary story is indeed an honor. I felt her spiritual presence by my side each day as I poured myself into its completion. Deborah's words, and her life, are a tribute to those professionals dealing with the alcohol and drug addiction population, as well as, those fighting the battle to be free from this population.

Howard Thurman, the infamous theologian, philosopher, and author of twenty books once wrote, "Don't ask yourself what the world needs. Ask yourself what makes you come alive, and go do that, because what the world needs is people who have come alive." I believe Deborah did exactly what kept her passion alive—guide those with drug addictions to recover their self-worth and find freedom in sobriety. She continued counseling even while undergoing radiation therapy, chemotherapy, and the loss of her hair. Deborah was an example of the bravery she instilled in her clients, she died in the spring of 2006.

In his later years, Aldous Huxley, who wrote many books questioning our world's view became a noted screenwriter with many films to his credit. He, like Deborah, strove to write with a sense of sincerity to expand our view of society. One of Huxley's most famous books, *Brave New World*, instilled surprise, disbelief, and unending questioning from its readers. Deborah and I hope this book has done the same for you.

Deborah shared with me that she wanted her manuscript to be made into a screenplay one day. I know if Huxley were alive today, he would find within these pages the perfect vase to hold a bouquet of words in which to produce a play that would open the mind of society to investigate what is really going on within our addiction populated world. He once wrote in his later life, "It's a bit embarrassing to have been concerned with the human problem all one's life and find at the end that one has no more to offer (by way of advice) than this: Try to be a little kinder." I believe Deborah agrees completely.

Dr. Barbara (Dora) Sinor

Resources

Addiction Resource Guide
www.addictionresourceguide.com/directory.html

Addiction Treatment Forum
Phone 847-392-3937
www.ATForum.com

Advocates for the Integration of Recovery and Methadone (AFIRM)
Phone 516-897-1330
afirmfwc@aol.com

Alcoholics Anonymous®
Phone 212-870-3400
www.alcoholics-anonymous.org

American Association for the Treatment of Opioid Dependence (AA-TOD)
Phone 212-355-4647
www.aatod.org

American Council on Alcoholism
Phone 800-527-5344

www.aca-usa.org
American Council for Drug Education
800-488-DRUG
www.acde.org

American Society of Addiction Medicine (ASAM)
www.asam.org

Center for Alcohol & Addiction Studies at Brown University
Phone 401-863-6600
www.caas.brown.edu

Centers for Disease Control & Prevention (CDC)
800-CDC-INFO (800-232-4636)
www.cdc.gov

Center for Substance Abuse Treatment (CSAT)
Treatment Facility Locator
http://dasis3.samhsa.gov/

Center for Substance Abuse Prevention
(240) 276-2420
http://prevention.samhsa.gov

Drug & Crime Statistics
Office of Justice Programs
U.S. Department of Justice
202-307-0703

Drug Enforcement Administration (DEA)
202-307-1000
www.dea.gov

Faces & Voices of Recovery
202-737-0690
www.facesandvoicesofrecovery.org

Methadone Anonymous (MA)
http://www.methadone-anonymous.org

Narcotics Anonymous
www.na.org

National Alliance of Methadone Advocates (NAMA)
212-595-NAMA
nama.info@methadone.org

National Association of Alcohol, Drugs, & Disability (NAADD)
650-578.8047
www.naadd.org

National Association of Social Workers (NASW)
202-408-8600
www.socialworkers.org

National Association of State Alcohol & Drug Abuse Directors (NA-SADAD)
1025 Connecticut Avenue NW, Suite 605
Washington, DC 20036
202-293-0090

National Council on Alcoholism and Drug Dependence (NCADD)
244 East 58th Street, 4th Floor
New York, NY 10022
212/269-7797

National Institute on Alcohol Abuse and Alcoholism (NIAAA)
5635 Fishers Lane, MSC 9304
Bethesda, MD 20892-9304
301-443-3860

National Institute on Drug Abuse (NIDA)
6001 Executive Boulevard, Room 5213
Bethesda, MD 20892-9561

Opioid Treatment Program Directory
1 Choke Cherry Road, Room 2-1075
Rockville, MD 20857
240-276-2700
otp@samhsa.hhs.gov

SMART Recovery®
www.smartrecovery.org

Substance Abuse & Mental Health Services Administration (SAMHSA)
Health Information Network
www.samhsa.gov/shin

World Health Organization
http://www.who.int

About the Author

Barbara Sinor, PhD is a Psychospiritual Therapist working with individuals dealing with addictions, childhood abuse/incest, PTSD, and adult children of alcoholics. Barbara utilizes a holistic methodology in her counseling encompassing forms of hypnotherapy, regression therapy, Gestalt, Jungian dreamwork, and other transpersonal techniques.

Dr. Sinor holds a Doctorate in Psychology; a Master of Arts from John F. Kennedy University; and her Bachelor of Arts degree is from Pitzer College.

Coming Soon: *Tales of Addiction* which documents personal stories of drug and/or alcohol addiction.

Dr. Sinor encourages your comments and can be contacted through her web site at www.DrSinor.com or write to: P.O. Box 382 Middletown, CA 95461.

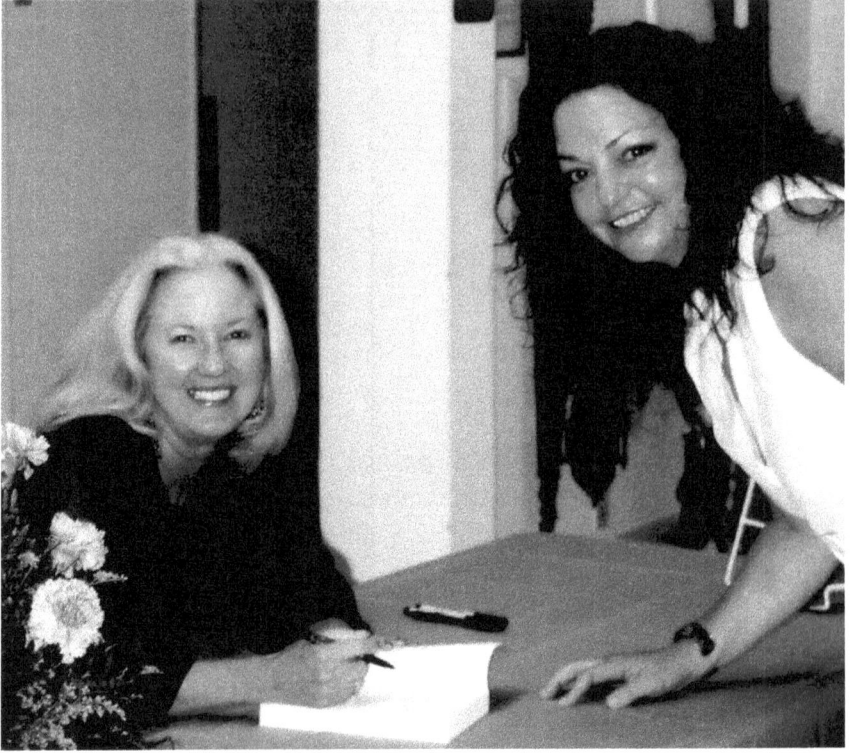

Barbara Sinor (left) with Deborah McCloskey (right) in 2004

Bibliography

Ashton, R. *This is heroin*. London: Sanctuary Publishing Limited, 2002.

Booth, L. Father. *Say yes to your spirit: A personal journey for developing spirituality, recovery, and healing*. Florida: Health Communications, Inc., 2008.

Fernandez, H. *Heroin*. Minnesota: Hazelden, 1998.

Henningfield, J. E., Santora, P. B., & Bickel, W. K. (2007). *Addiction treatment: Science and policy for the twenty-first century*. Baltimore: Johns Hopkins University Press.

Hoffman, J.; Froemke, S., Cheever, S.; and Nevins, S. *Addiction: Why Can't They Just Stop*. New York: Rodale Books, 2007.

Lydon, S.G. *Take the long way home*. California: HarperSanFrancisco, 1994.

McCoy, A.W. *The politics of heroin: CIA complicity in the global drug trade*. Illinois: Lawrence Hill Books, 2003.

Moreas, F. *The heroin user's handbook*. Washington: Loompanics Unlimited, 2004.

Peele, S. *The meaning of addiction: an unconventional view*. California: Jossey-Bass, Inc., 1998.

Peele, S., Brodsky, A., & Arnold, M. (1991). *The truth about addiction and recovery: The life process program for outgrowing destructive habits*. New York: Simon & Schuster.

Schneider, E. C. (2008). *Smack: Heroin and the American city*. Politics and culture in modern America. Philadelphia: University of Pennsylvania Press.

Seivewright, N., & Parry, M. (2009). *Community treatment of drug misuse: More than methadone.* New York: Cambridge University Press.

Smethers, J. *Scumbag sewer rats: An archetypal understanding of criminalized drug addicts.* Ireland: CheckPoint Press, 2008.

Snyder, S. H. (1986). *Drugs and the brain.* Scientific American Library series, no. 18. New York: Scientific American Books.

Steven L.; Janice F. Kauffman; Ira Marion; Mark W. Parrino; George E. and Woody Batki. (2006) *Medication Assisted Treatment for Opioid Addiction in Opioid Treatment Programs* TIP 43. SAMHSA: U.S. Department of Health and Human Servicse.

Strain, E. C., & Stitzer, M. L. (2006). *The treatment of opioid dependence.* Baltimore: Johns Hopkins University Press.

Volpicelli, J. *Recovery options: the complete guide.* New York: John Wiley & Sons, Inc., 2000.

Ward, J., Mattick, R. P., & Hall, W. (1998). *Methadone maintenance treatment and other opioid replacement therapies.* Amsterdam: Harwood Academic.

Wechsberg, W. M., & Kasten, J. J. (2007). *Methadone maintenance treatment in the U.S.: A practical question and answer guide.* New York: Springer.

Weil, A., & Rosen, W. (1993). *From chocolate to morphine: Everything you need to know about mind-altering drugs.* Boston: Houghton Mifflin.

Wynn, G. H. (2009). *Clinical manual of drug interaction principles for medical practice.* Washington, DC: American Psychiatric Pub.

Index

Gifts From
The Child Within
Second Edition

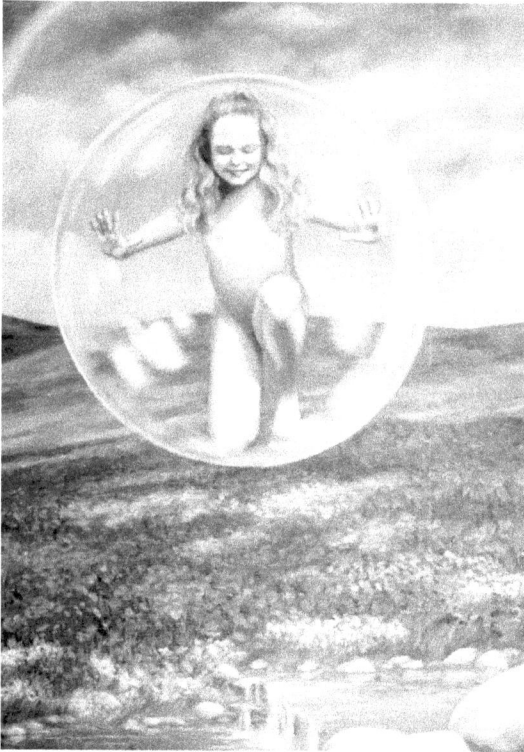

Barbara Sinor, PhD

"Gifts From The Child Within is more than a well-written, well-researched guide to recover from our childhood wounds. It is an exciting adventure in psychospiritual growth based on inner wisdom exercises that are a powerful addition to the archives of healing"

Joan Borysenko, PhD, Author of *Your Soul's Compass*